MOCKTAILS
for the
HOLIDAYS

NON-ALCOHOLIC DRINKS FOR
COZY AUTUMN NIGHTS AND WINTER FESTIVITIES

Book 6 of the Mocktails for Every Day Series

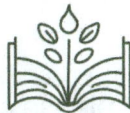

green sauce
— PUBLISHING —

TABLE OF CONTENTS

TABLE OF CONTENTS

TABLE OF CONTENTS

HOT CHOCOLATES & COZY DRINKS

HOMEMADE SYRUPS, CORDIALS, & INFUSIONS

Cheers to a Joyful Season!

There's something truly magical about the holidays. Whether you celebrate Christmas, Hanukkah, Kwanzaa, New Year, the Solstice—or simply enjoy the sparkle of the season—gatherings during this time are full of joy, generosity, and indulgence. But here's the thing: you don't need alcohol to celebrate in style. That's where mocktails come in.

Why Mocktails?

Mocktails bring the sparkle without the spirits. They're inclusive, delicious, and suitable for everyone at the party—kids, pregnant friends, designated drivers, health-conscious guests, and those avoiding alcohol for any reason at all.

Holiday mocktails in particular are something special. Think cozy spices, vibrant cranberries, fresh citrus, warming infusions, and beautiful garnishes. They don't just taste good—they feel like a celebration in a glass.

Whether you're hosting a festive brunch, bringing a pitcher to a potluck, or snuggling by the fire with a good book, a holiday mocktail can add a little extra magic to the moment.

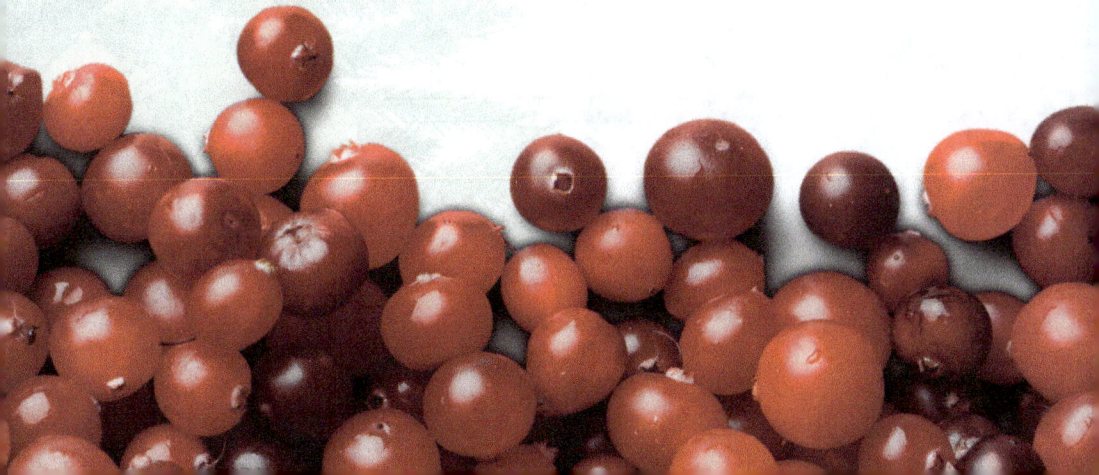

What You'll Need

Just like the other books in the Mocktails for Every Day series, this one is designed to be easy, accessible, and joyful. You won't need fancy bartending skills or hard-to-find ingredients.

Here's a quick overview of the basic tools and ingredients that will come in handy:

- A good citrus juicer or reamer – fresh juice makes all the difference.

- A strainer or sieve – useful for removing pulp or spice bits.

- Jars or bottles – for storing homemade syrups and infusions.

- A saucepan – for making simple syrups and warming drinks.

- A cocktail shaker or large mason jar with a lid – perfect for blending flavors.

- Spoons and jugs for stirring and serving.

- Optional: A blender or stick blender – for frothy drinks and smooth blends.

- Pretty glassware – because presentation counts, especially during the holidays!

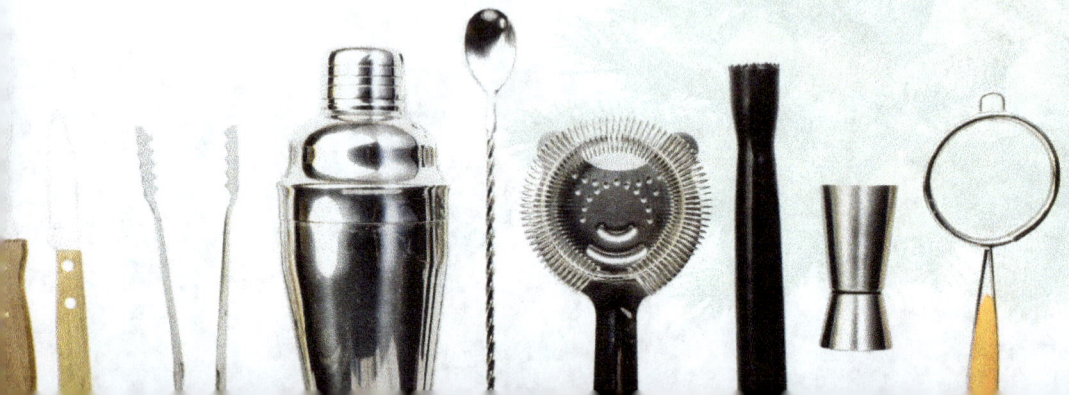

Ingredients

You'll find many of the ingredients in this book at your local supermarket or already in your pantry or fridge. We keep things seasonal, simple, and delicious.

Common stars include:

- Fresh citrus fruits like oranges, lemons, limes, and grapefruit.

- Berries (especially cranberries), pomegranate, apple, and pear.

- Herbs and spices like cinnamon, clove, rosemary, thyme, star anise, nutmeg, and ginger.

- Syrups and cordials—many of which can be homemade using recipes from Book 3 (Mocktail Syrups and Flavors).

- Sparkling water, soda water, or non-alcoholic sparkling wine for fizz.

- Dairy-free milks, such as oat, almond, or coconut, for creamy holiday treats.

And of course, ice, citrus zest, and festive garnishes to bring it all together.

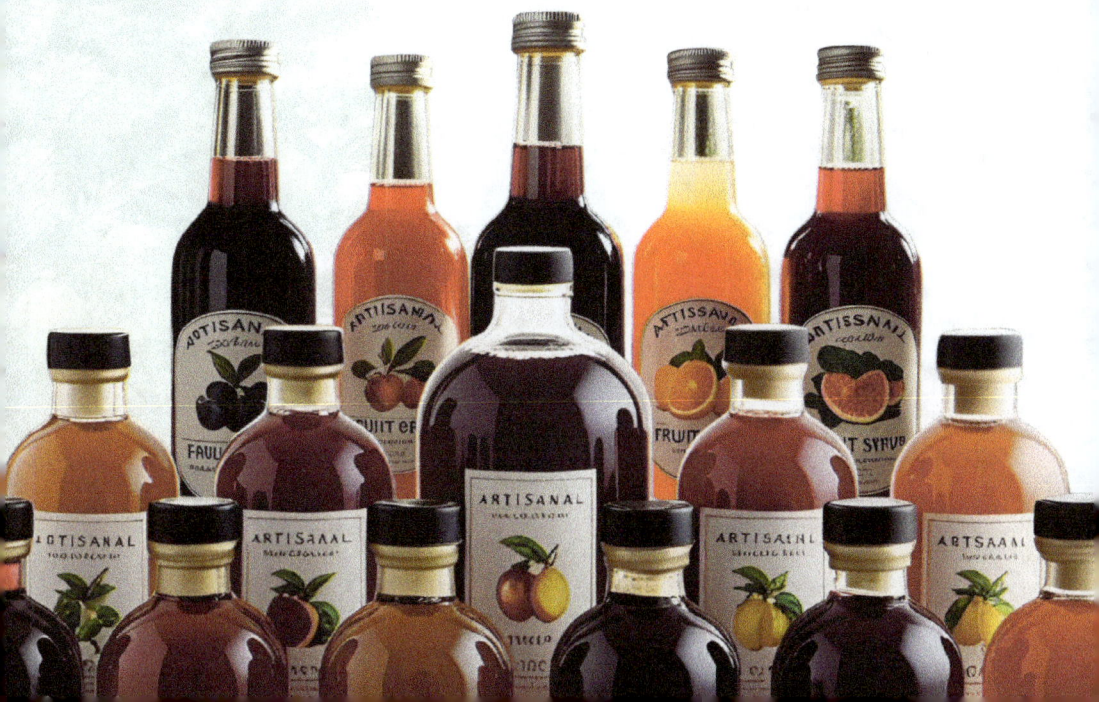

Homemade with Love

As always, this book includes a mix of quick-and-easy recipes and more elaborate showstoppers. You'll also find tips for making ahead, batch-serving, and creating beautiful presentations with minimal effort.

Each recipe is alcohol-free, family-friendly, and designed to serve four people. You can easily double or halve the quantities depending on your gathering.

Let's Get Festive

The holidays can be chaotic, busy, and emotional—so having a joyful, comforting drink in your hand can be a small but meaningful way to pause, connect, and celebrate.

Whether you're raising a glass with loved ones or enjoying a quiet night by the fire, these mocktails are here to make your holidays a little more delicious.

Let's toast to the season—with warmth, gratitude, and something wonderful in your glass.

Cheers!

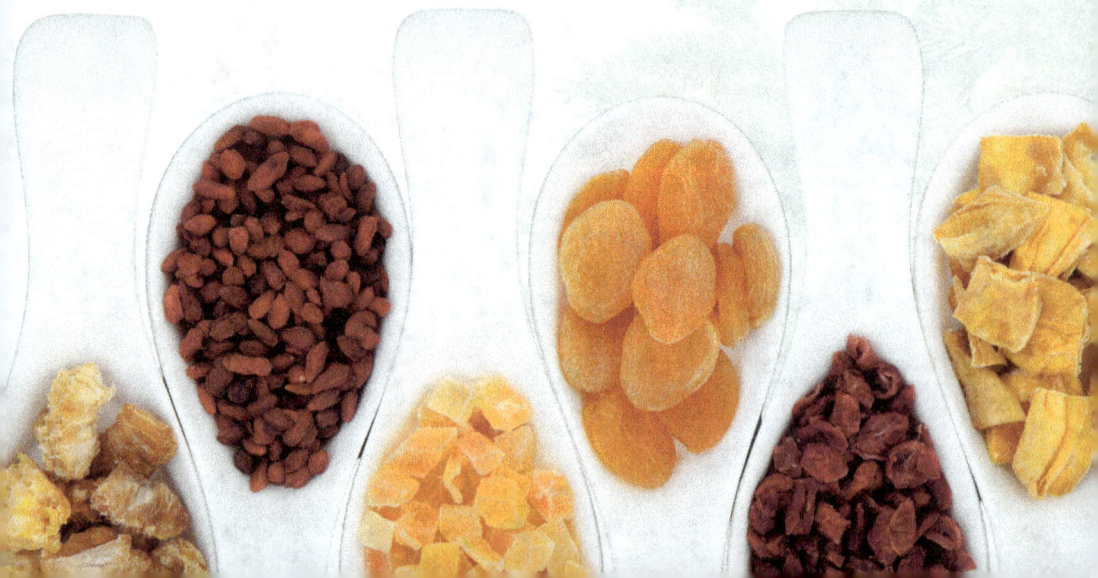

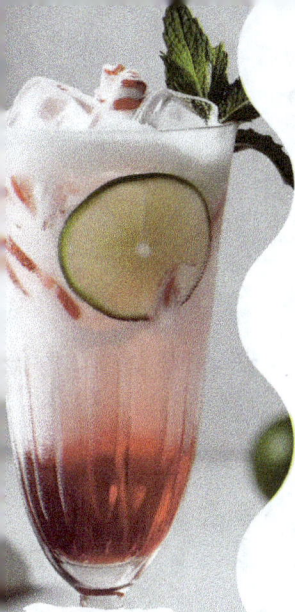

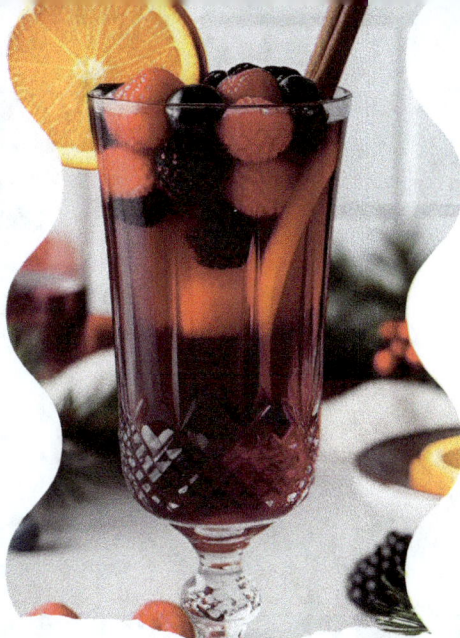

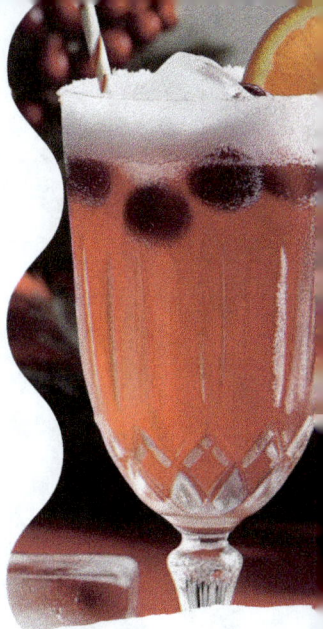

CLASSIC CHRISTMAS MOCKTAILS

These classic Christmas mocktails are festive, flavorful, and perfect for holiday gatherings.

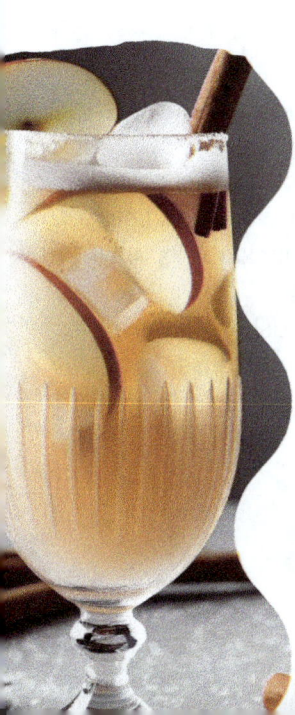

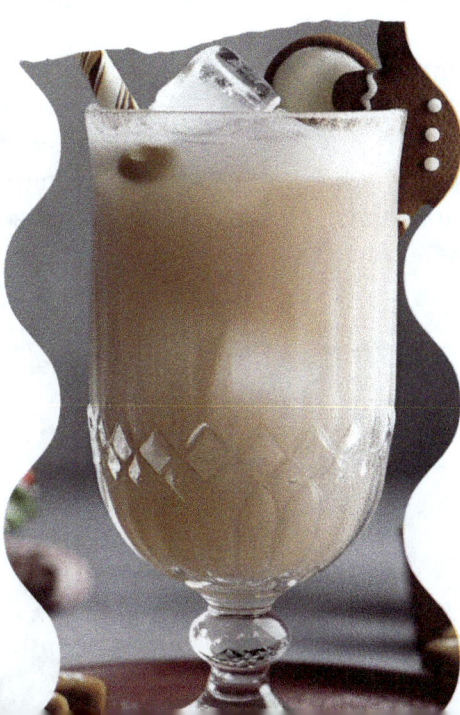

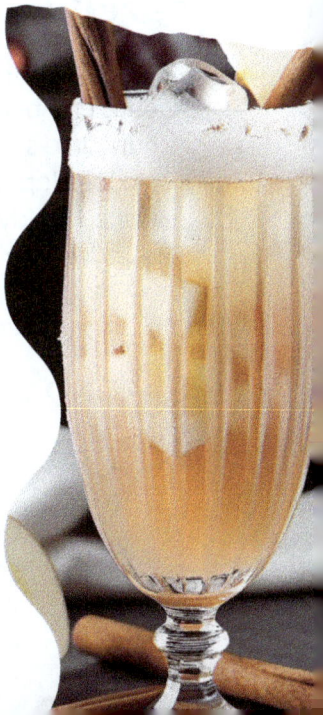

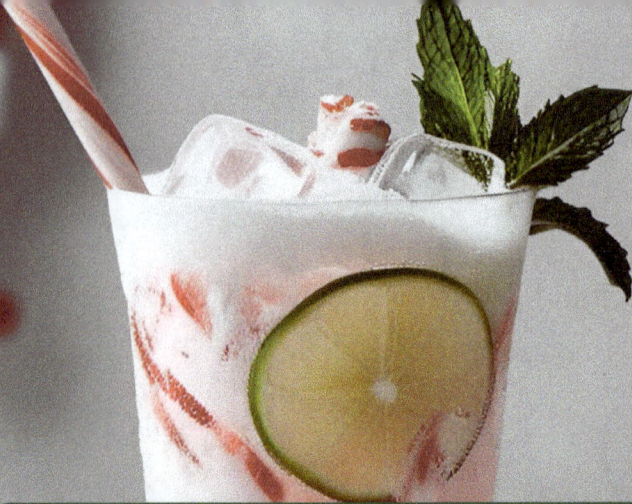

Candy Cane Cooler

Like sipping a Christmas candy cane—cool, minty, and festively fun with a cranberry twist.

Serving Size	Serving Time
4 people	10 min.

Ingredients

- 1/2 cup peppermint syrup
- 2 cups cranberry juice
- 3 cups lime soda
- Ice cubes (optional)
- Crushed candy canes and mint leaves for garnish

Procedure

1. In a pitcher, combine the peppermint syrup and cranberry juice. Stir well.
2. Add the lime soda and stir gently.
3. Fill four glasses with ice (if using) and pour the mocktail mixture into the glasses.
4. Garnish with crushed candy canes and mint leaves before serving.

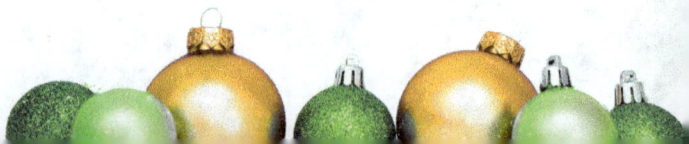

Spiced Apple Cider Fizz

A bubbly blend of apple cider and cinnamon that brings the holiday cheer in every sparkling sip.

Serving Size	Serving Time
4 people	10 min.

Ingredients

- 2 cups fresh apple cider
- 1/2 cup cinnamon syrup
- 3 cups club soda
- Ice cubes (optional)
- Cinnamon sticks and apple slices for garnish

Procedure

1. In a pitcher, combine the fresh apple cider and cinnamon syrup. Stir well.
2. Add the club soda and stir gently to mix.
3. Fill four glasses with ice (if using) and pour the mocktail mixture into the glasses.
4. Garnish with cinnamon sticks and apple slices before serving.

Cranberry Orange Sparkler

Zingy citrus meets tart cranberry for a merry and bright refreshment.

Serving Size	Serving Time
4 people	10 min.

Ingredients

- 2 cups fresh cranberry juice
- 1/2 cup orange cordial
- 3 cups sparkling water
- Ice cubes (optional)
- Orange slices and cranberries for garnish

Procedure

1. In a pitcher, combine the cranberry juice and orange cordial. Stir well.
2. Add the sparkling water and stir gently.
3. Fill four glasses with ice (if using) and pour the mocktail mixture into the glasses.
4. Garnish with orange slices and cranberries before serving.

Gingerbread Punch

Cozy up with this creamy delight that tastes just like a freshly baked gingerbread cookie.

Serving Size	Serving Time
4 people	10 min.

Ingredients

- 1/2 cup gingerbread syrup
- 2 cups almond milk
- 1 teaspoon vanilla extract
- Ice cubes (optional)
- Freshly grated nutmeg and gingerbread cookies for garnish

Procedure

1. In a pitcher, combine the gingerbread syrup, almond milk, and vanilla extract. Stir well.
2. Fill four glasses with ice (if using) and pour the punch into the glasses.
3. Garnish with freshly grated nutmeg and a gingerbread cookie on the rim before serving.

Mulled Berry Mocktail

A warm and comforting berry hug spiced with holiday magic—perfect for chilly nights.

Serving Size	Serving Time
4 people	10 min.

Ingredients

- 2 cups mixed berry juice (from blueberries, raspberries, and blackberries)
- 1/2 cup mulling spice infusion
- 1 cup water
- Orange slices for garnish

Procedure

1. In a saucepan, combine the berry juice, mulling spice infusion, and water. Heat over medium heat until warm (do not boil).
2. Remove from heat and let it sit for a few minutes to fully infuse.
3. Pour the mixture into four heatproof glasses.
4. Garnish with orange slices before serving.

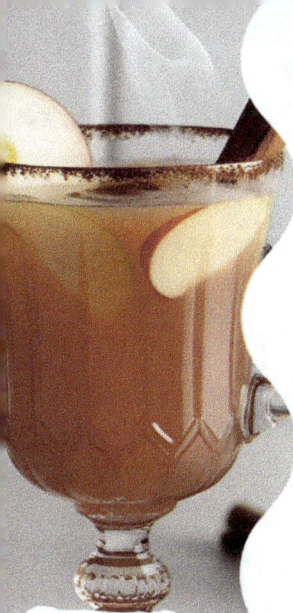

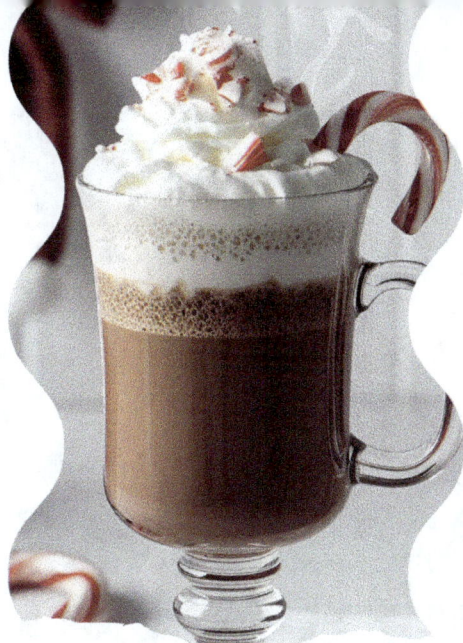

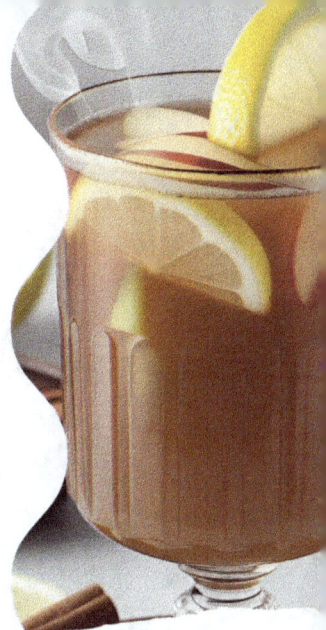

COZY WARM WINTER MOCKTAILS

These cozy warm winter mocktails are perfect for staying warm during the holiday season.

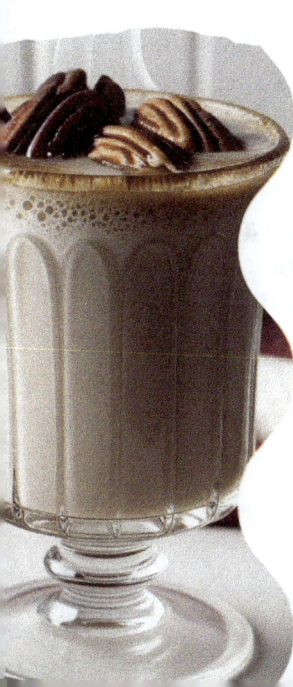

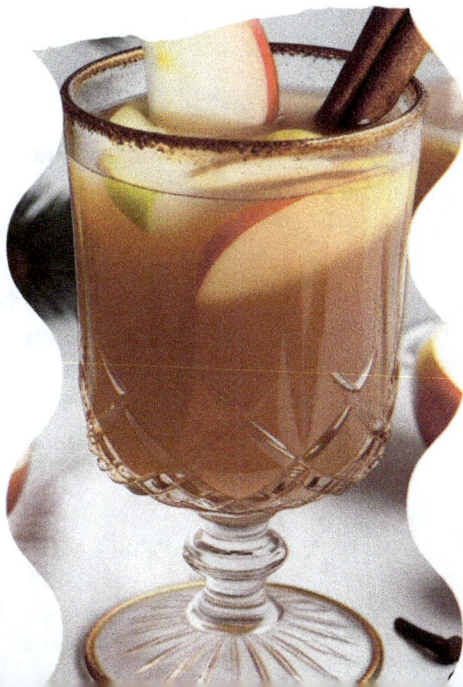

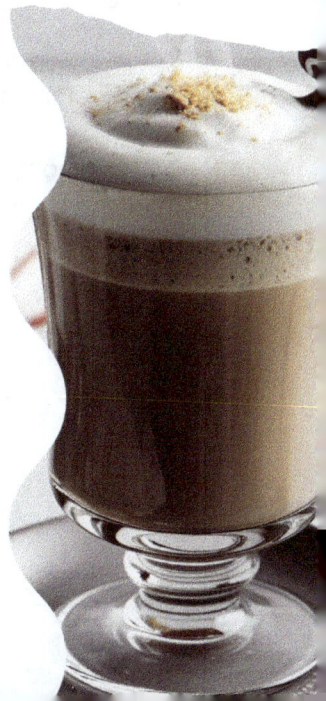

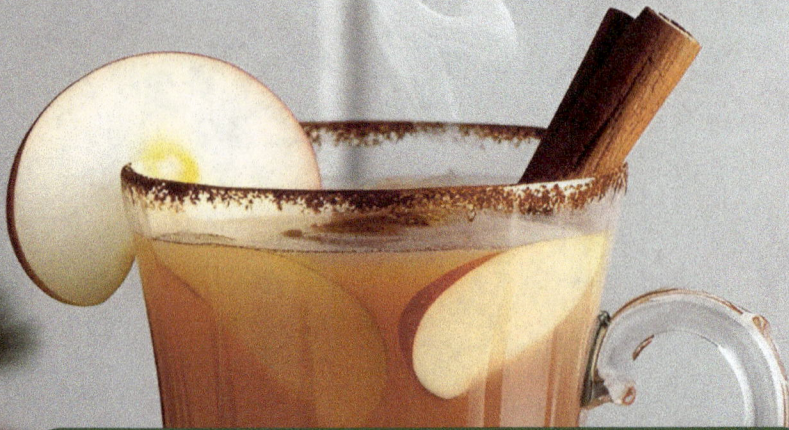

Hot Spiced Cinnamon Punch

A steaming mug of apple and spice—like a cozy blanket for your tastebuds.

Serving Size	Serving Time
4 people	10 min.

Ingredients

- 3 cups fresh apple juice
- 1/2 cup cinnamon syrup (recipe below)
- 1/2 teaspoon ground cloves
- Cinnamon sticks and apple slices for garnish

Procedure

1. In a saucepan, combine the apple juice, cinnamon syrup, and ground cloves.
2. Heat over medium-low heat until the mixture is warm (do not boil).
3. Remove from heat and let it sit for a few minutes to infuse the flavors.
4. Pour into four heatproof mugs.
5. Garnish each mug with a cinnamon stick and an apple slice before serving.

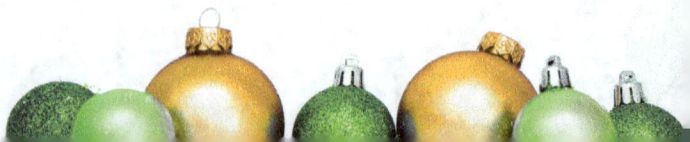

Warm Peppermint Hot Chocolate

Minty, chocolatey, and rich—this one's like a warm hug from the North Pole.

Serving Size	Serving Time
4 people	10 min.

Ingredients

- 3 cups almond milk (or any milk of your choice)
- 1/2 cup cocoa powder
- 1/2 cup peppermint infusion
- 1 teaspoon vanilla extract
- Whipped cream and crushed candy canes for garnish

Procedure

1. In a saucepan, warm the almond milk over medium heat. Whisk in the cocoa powder until well combined.
2. Add the peppermint infusion and vanilla extract, stirring until warm (do not boil).
3. Pour into four heatproof mugs.
4. Top each mug with whipped cream and crushed candy canes before serving.

Toasty Maple Pecan Delight

Nutty, sweet, and irresistibly warming—maple and pecan are a perfect winter pair.

Serving Size	Serving Time
4 people	10 min.

Ingredients

- 3 cups toasted pecan milk
- 1/4 cup maple syrup
- 1/2 teaspoon ground cinnamon
- 1/4 teaspoon ground nutmeg
- Toasted pecans and a cinnamon stick for garnish

Procedure

1. In a saucepan, warm the toasted pecan milk over medium heat. Stir in the maple syrup, ground cinnamon, and nutmeg.
2. Heat until the mixture is warm (do not boil).
3. Pour into four heatproof mugs.

Chai Spiced Apple Toddy

Bold chai meets sweet apple in this soul-warming twist on tradition.

Serving Size	Serving Time
4 people	10 min.

Ingredients

- 3 cups fresh apple juice
- 1/2 cup chai syrup
- 1 tablespoon fresh lemon juice
- Cinnamon sticks and lemon slices for garnish

Procedure

1. In a saucepan, combine the apple juice, chai syrup, and lemon juice. Heat over medium-low heat until warm (do not boil).
2. Pour the mixture into four heatproof mugs.
3. Garnish each mug with a cinnamon stick and a lemon slice before serving.

Gingerbread Latte Mocktail

The nostalgic flavor of gingerbread meets your favorite cozy latte—no caffeine crash here!

Serving Size	Serving Time
4 people	10 min.

Ingredients

- 2 cups brewed coffee (cooled slightly)
- 1/2 cup gingerbread syrup (recipe from section 1)
- 2 cups frothed almond milk (or any milk of your choice)
- Freshly grated nutmeg for garnish

Procedure

1. In a saucepan, warm the brewed coffee and gingerbread syrup over medium heat until warm.
2. Divide the mixture into four heatproof mugs.
3. Top each mug with frothed almond milk.
4. Garnish with freshly grated nutmeg before serving.

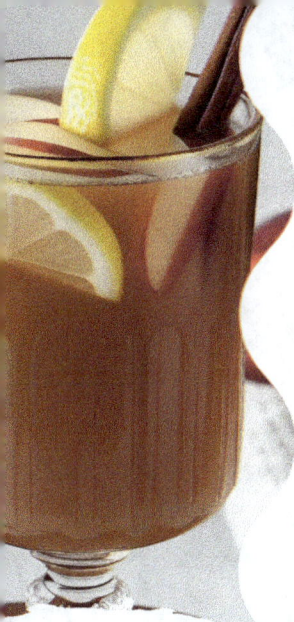

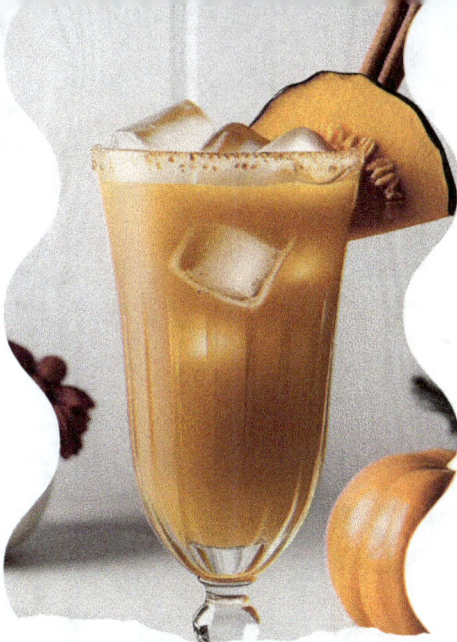

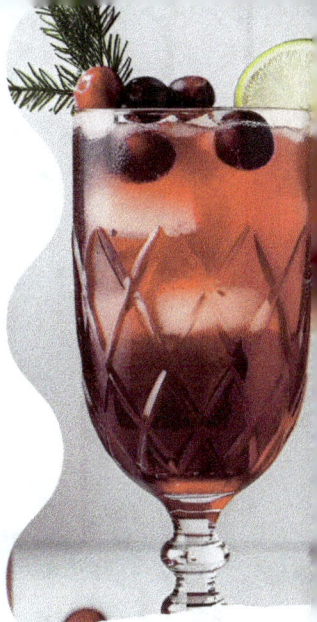

THANKSGIVING FAVORITES

These Thanksgiving mocktails bring seasonal flavors to the forefront, perfect for celebrating with friends and family.

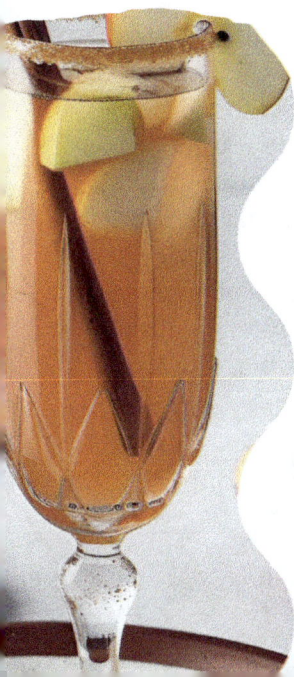

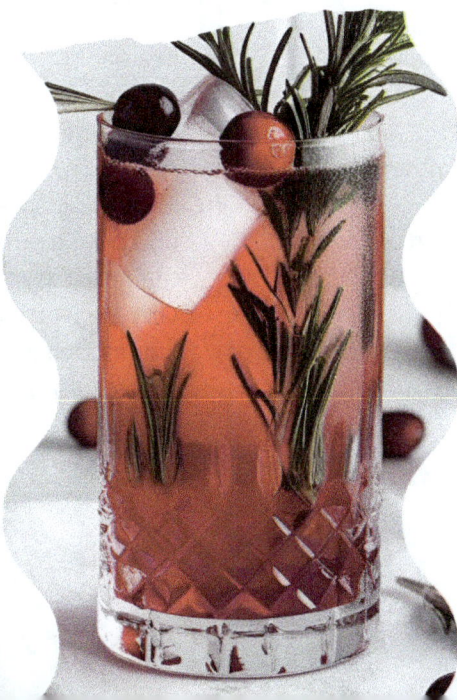

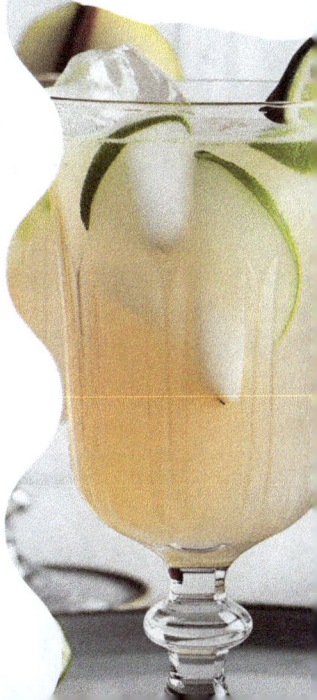

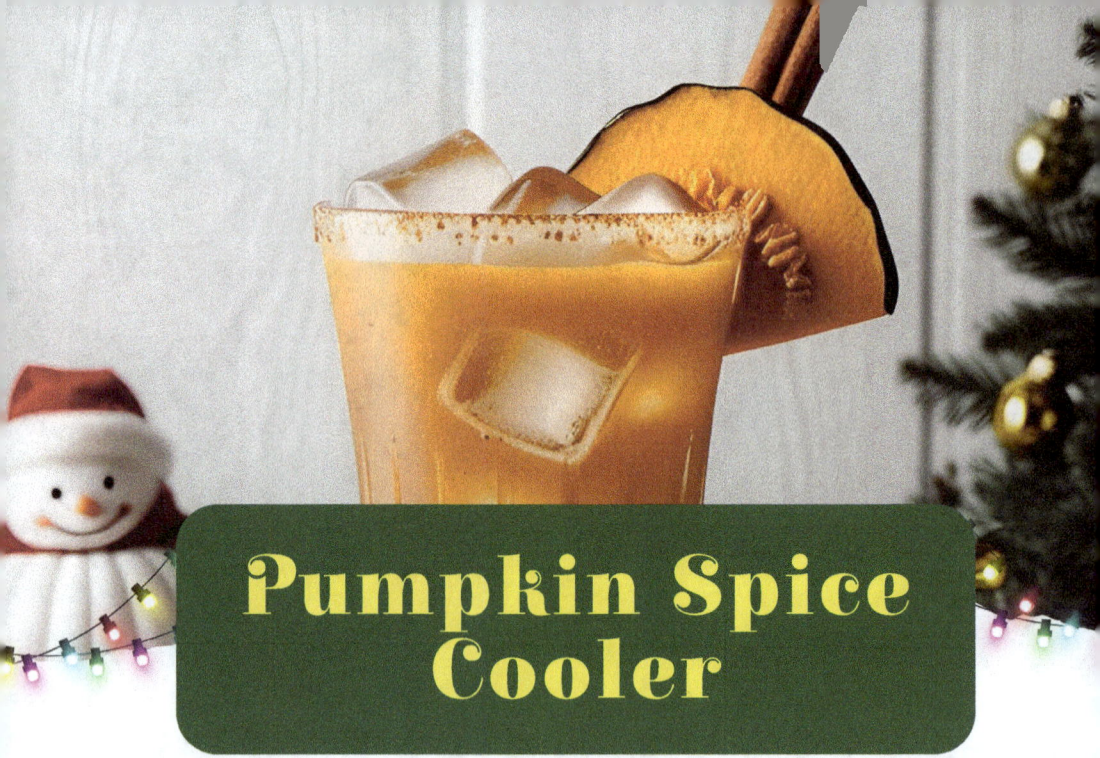

Pumpkin Spice Cooler

Cool, creamy, and full of pumpkin pie vibes—Thanksgiving in a glass.

Serving Size	Serving Time
4 people	10 min.

Ingredients

- 1/2 cup pumpkin puree
- 1/2 cup cinnamon syrup
- 3 cups club soda
- Dash of ground nutmeg
- Ice cubes (optional)
- Cinnamon sticks and pumpkin slices for garnish

Procedure

1. In a pitcher, whisk together the pumpkin puree and cinnamon syrup until well combined.
2. Add the club soda and stir gently.
3. Fill four glasses with ice (if using) and pour the mocktail mixture into the glasses.
4. Garnish with a dash of nutmeg, cinnamon sticks, and pumpkin slices before serving.

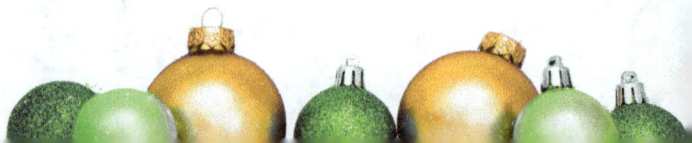

Cranberry Rosemary Spritz

Elegant and earthy with a touch of sparkle—perfect for a festive toast.

Serving Size	Serving Time
4 people	10 min.

Ingredients

- 2 cups fresh cranberry juice
- 1/2 cup rosemary syrup
- 3 cups sparkling water
- Ice cubes (optional)
- Fresh rosemary sprigs and cranberries for garnish

Procedure

1. In a pitcher, combine the cranberry juice and rosemary syrup. Stir well.
2. Add the sparkling water and stir gently.
3. Fill four glasses with ice (if using) and pour the mocktail mixture into the glasses.
4. Garnish with fresh rosemary sprigs and cranberries before serving.

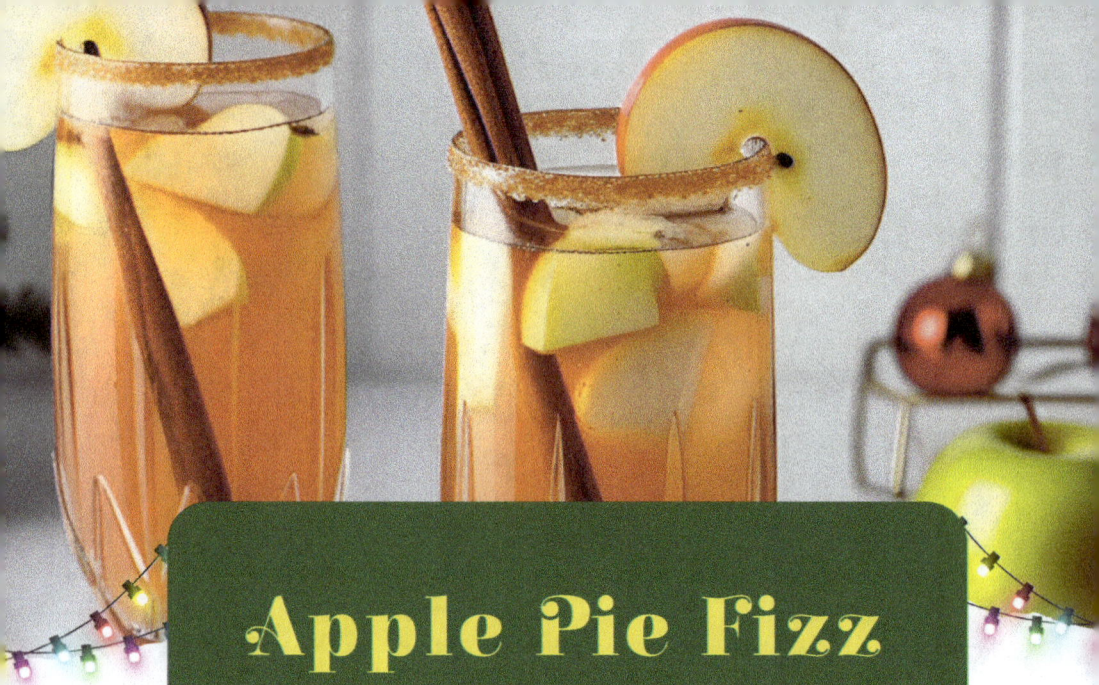

Apple Pie Fizz

Just like grandma's pie, only fizzy—with a hint of cinnamon sugar on the rim.

Serving Size	Serving Time
4 people	10 min.

Ingredients

- 2 cups fresh apple cider
- 1/2 cup cinnamon infusion
- 3 cups soda water
- Cinnamon sugar for rim
- Ice cubes (optional)
- Cinnamon sticks and apple slices for garnish

Procedure

1. To prepare the glasses, dip the rims in water and then coat with cinnamon sugar.
2. In a pitcher, combine the apple cider and cinnamon infusion. Stir well.
3. Add the soda water and stir gently.
4. Fill four glasses with ice (if using) and pour the mocktail mixture into the glasses.
5. Garnish with cinnamon sticks and apple slices before serving.

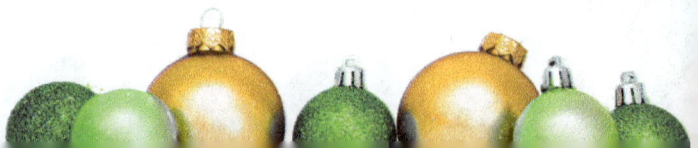

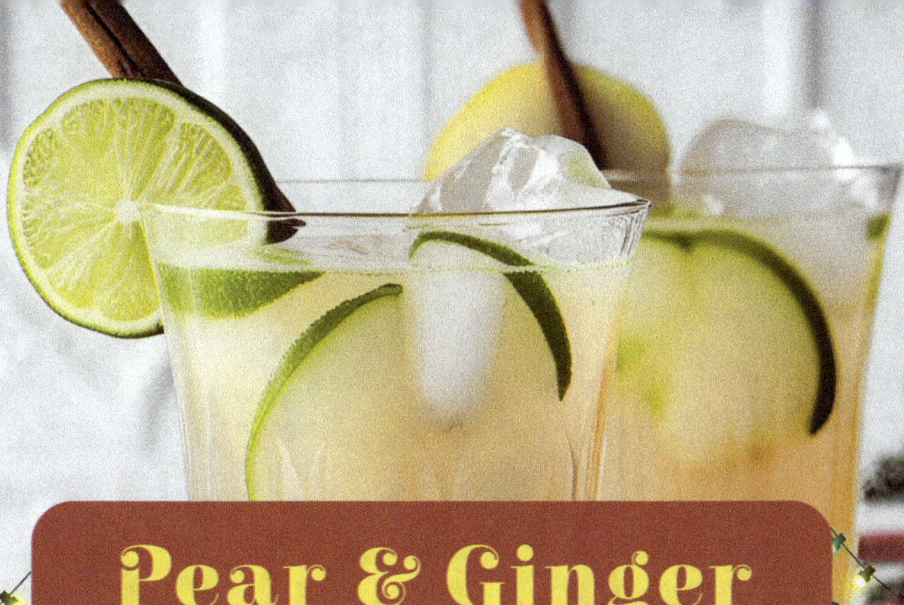

Pear & Ginger Punch

Light, spicy, and totally unexpected—an autumnal stunner in every glass.

Serving Size	Serving Time
4 people	10 min.

Ingredients

- 2 cups fresh pear juice (from about 4 ripe pears, pureed and strained)
- 1/2 cup ginger syrup
- 3 cups lime soda
- Ice cubes (optional)
- Fresh pear slices and lime wedges for garnish

Procedure

1. In a pitcher, combine the pear juice and ginger syrup. Stir well.
2. Add the lime soda and stir gently.
3. Fill four glasses with ice (if using) and pour the mocktail mixture into the glasses.
4. Garnish with fresh pear slices and lime wedges before serving.

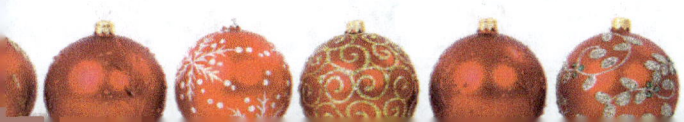

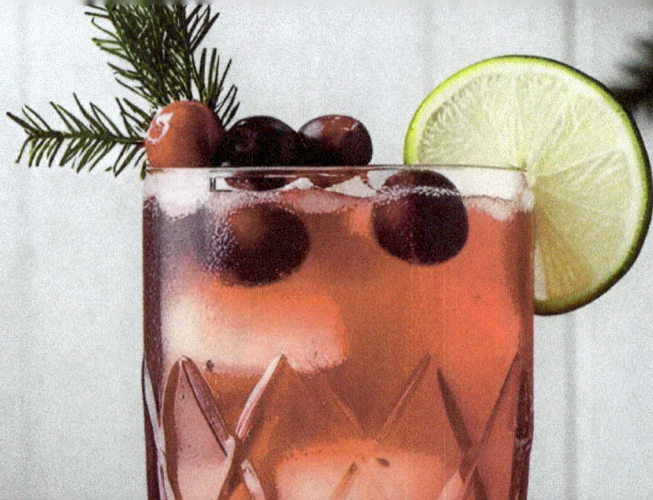

Spiced Cranberry Mule

A tangy, gingery twist on a classic—served icy cold in a copper mug.

Serving Size	Serving Time
4 people	10 min.

Ingredients

- 2 cups fresh cranberry juice
- 1/2 cup ginger syrup
- 3 cups lime soda
- Ice cubes
- Fresh lime slices and cranberries for garnish

Procedure

1. In a pitcher, combine the cranberry juice and ginger syrup. Stir well.
2. Add the lime soda and stir gently.
3. Fill four copper mugs or glasses with ice and pour the mocktail mixture into the glasses.
4. Garnish with lime slices and fresh cranberries before serving.

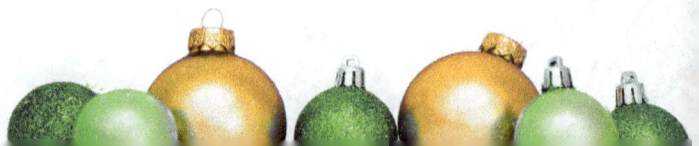

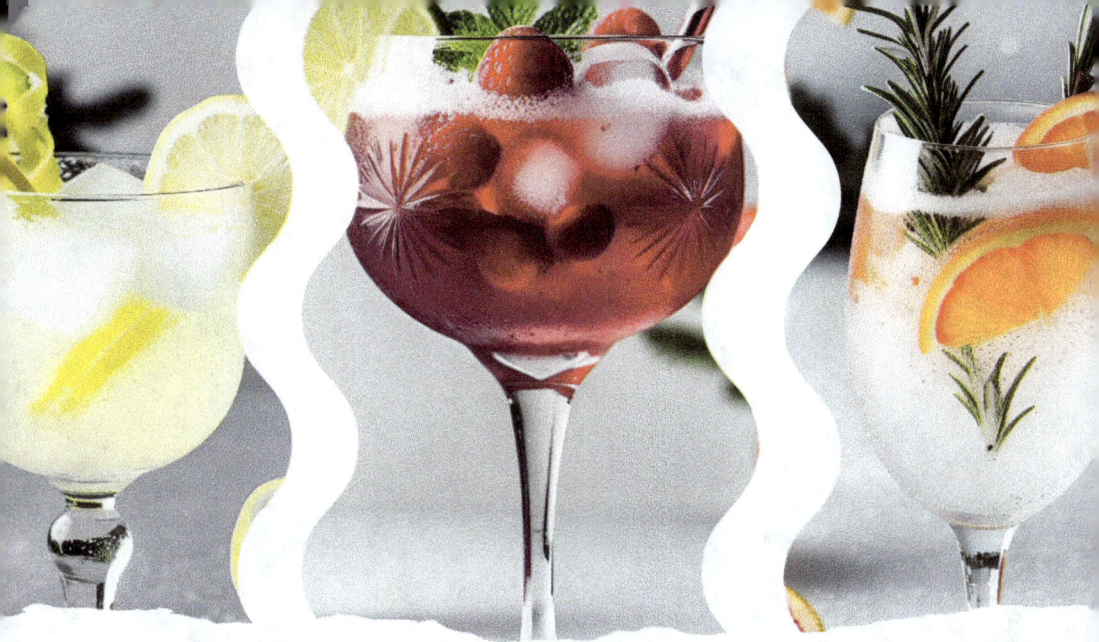

FESTIVE CITRUS MOCKTAILS

These festive citrus mocktails are bright and refreshing, perfect for adding a zesty touch to your holiday celebrations

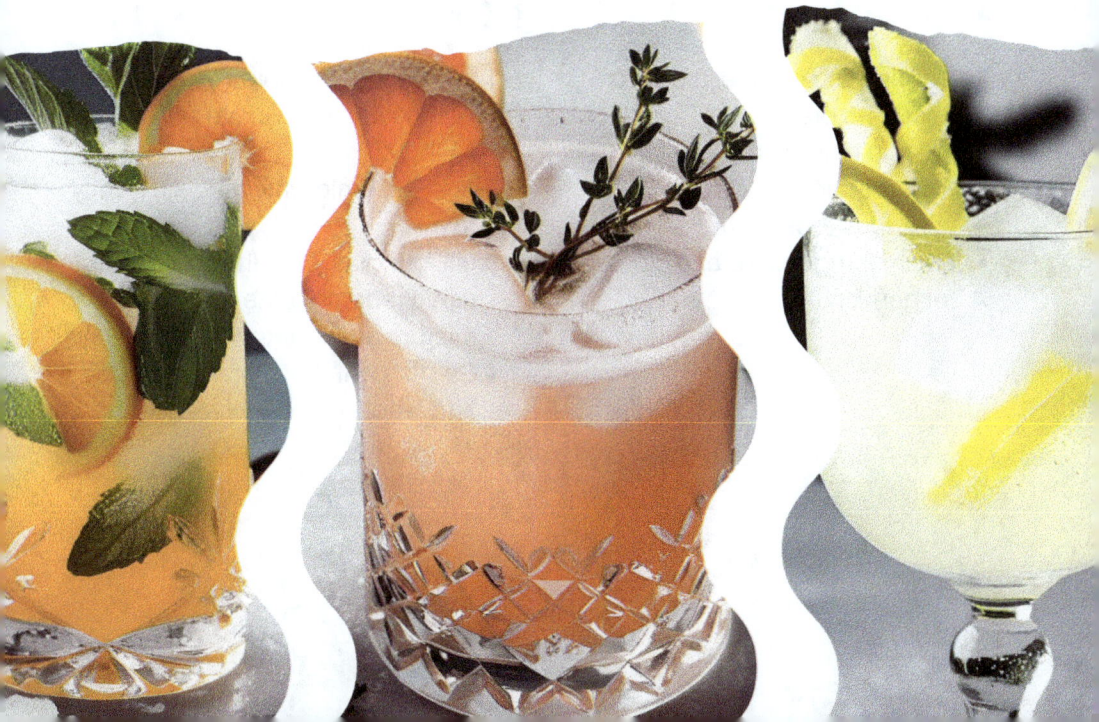

Orange Clove Sparkler

Bright orange and warm clove unite in this dazzling and delicious winter sparkler.

Serving Size	Serving Time
4 people	10 min.

Ingredients

- 2 cups fresh orange juice (from about 4-5 oranges)
- 1/2 cup clove syrup
- 3 cups tonic water
- Ice cubes (optional)
- Fresh orange slices and cloves for garnish

Procedure

1. In a pitcher, combine the fresh orange juice and clove syrup. Stir well.
2. Add the tonic water and stir gently to mix.
3. Fill four glasses with ice cubes (if using) and pour the mocktail mixture evenly into the glasses.
4. Garnish with fresh orange slices and whole cloves before serving.

Winter Citrus Spritz

A refreshing burst of blood orange with herbaceous flair—sunshine in every sip.

Serving Size	Serving Time
4 people	10 min.

Ingredients

- 2 cups fresh blood orange juice (from about 4-5 blood oranges)
- 1/2 cup rosemary infusion
- 3 cups sparkling water
- Ice cubes (optional)
- Fresh rosemary sprigs and blood orange slices for garnish

Procedure

1. In a pitcher, combine the blood orange juice and rosemary infusion. Stir well.
2. Add the sparkling water and stir gently.
3. Fill four glasses with ice (if using) and pour the mocktail mixture into the glasses.
4. Garnish with fresh rosemary sprigs and blood orange slices before serving.

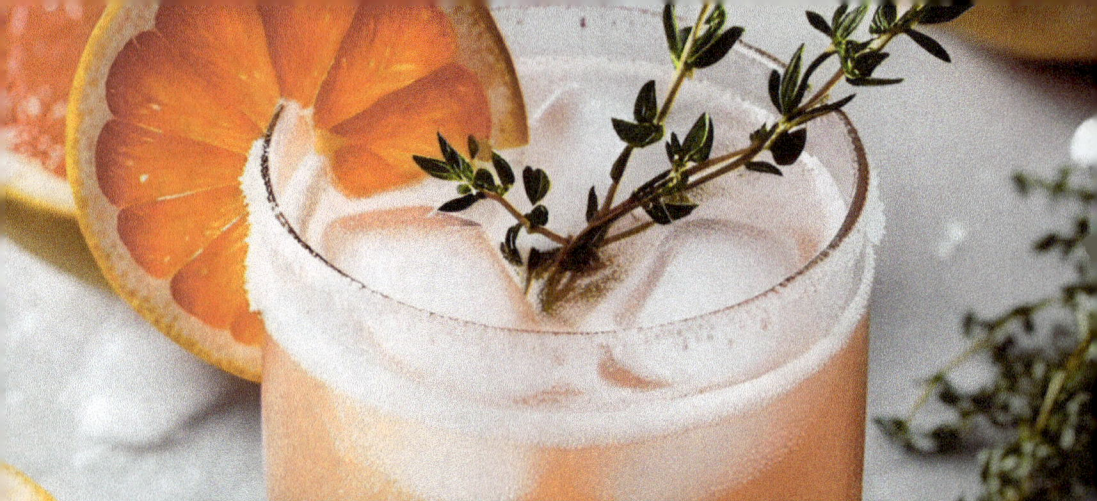

Grapefruit & Thyme Fizz

Zesty, herbal, and ever so chic—this one's a party pleaser with pizzazz.

Serving Size	Serving Time
4 people	10 min.

Ingredients

- 2 cups fresh grapefruit juice (from about 2 large grapefruits)
- 1/2 cup thyme syrup
- 3 cups soda water
- Ice cubes (optional)
- Fresh thyme sprigs and grapefruit slices for garnish

Procedure

1. In a pitcher, combine the grapefruit juice and thyme syrup. Stir well.
2. Add the soda water and stir gently.
3. Fill four glasses with ice (if using) and pour the mocktail mixture into the glasses.
4. Garnish with fresh thyme sprigs and grapefruit slices before serving.

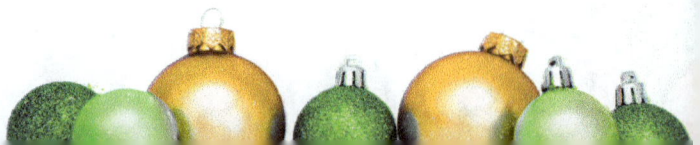

Lemon Ginger Zest

Lively and zingy, with a ginger kick that keeps the chill at bay.

Serving Size	Serving Time
4 people	10 min.

Ingredients

- 1 cup fresh lemon juice (from about 4-5 lemons)
- 1/2 cup ginger syrup
- 3 cups sparkling water
- Ice cubes (optional)
- Fresh lemon twists and ginger slices for garnish

Procedure

1. In a pitcher, combine the lemon juice and ginger syrup. Stir well.
2. Add the sparkling water and stir gently.
3. Fill four glasses with ice (if using) and pour the mocktail mixture into the glasses.
4. Garnish with lemon twists and ginger slices before serving.

Mandarin Mint Cooler

Sweet mandarin and cool mint combine for a refreshingly festive treat.

Serving Size	Serving Time
4 people	10 min.

Ingredients

- 2 cups fresh mandarin juice (from about 6-8 mandarins)
- 1/2 cup mint syrup
- 3 cups soda water
- Ice cubes (optional)
- Fresh mint leaves and mandarin slices for garnish

Procedure

1. In a pitcher, combine the mandarin juice and mint syrup. Stir well.
2. Add the soda water and stir gently.
3. Fill four glasses with ice (if using) and pour the mocktail mixture into the glasses.
4. Garnish with fresh mint leaves and mandarin slices before serving.

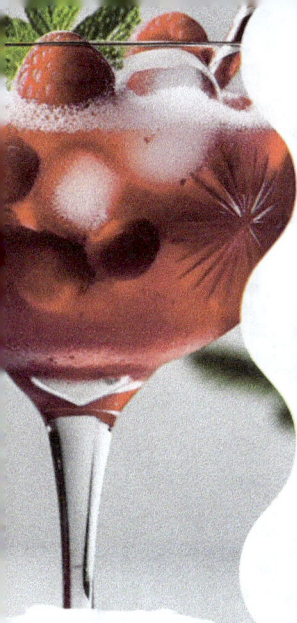

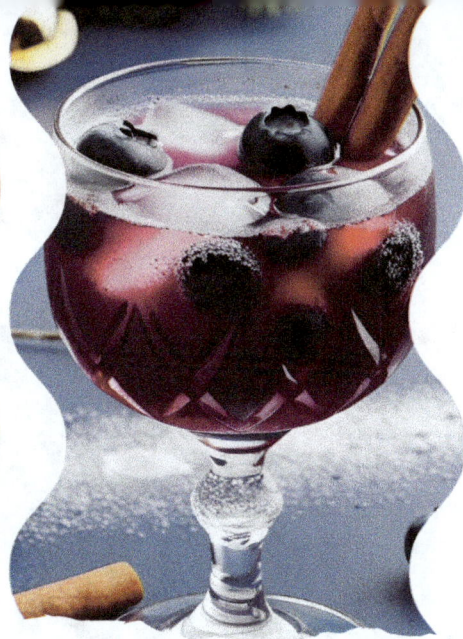

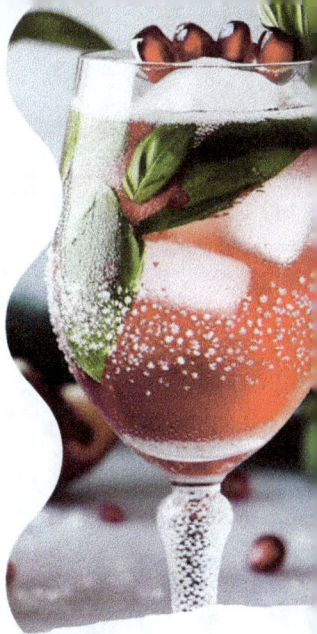

BERRY & POMEGRANATE DELIGHTS

These berry and pomegranate mocktails are vibrant, flavorful, and perfect for winter holiday celebrations.

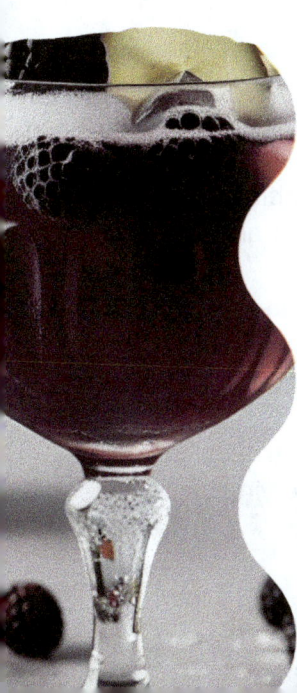

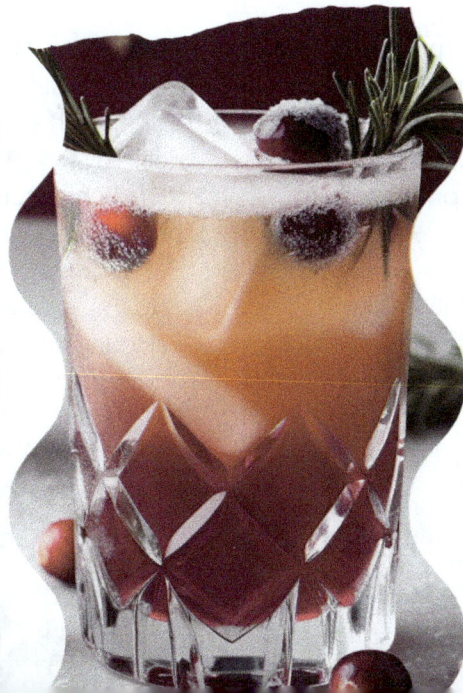

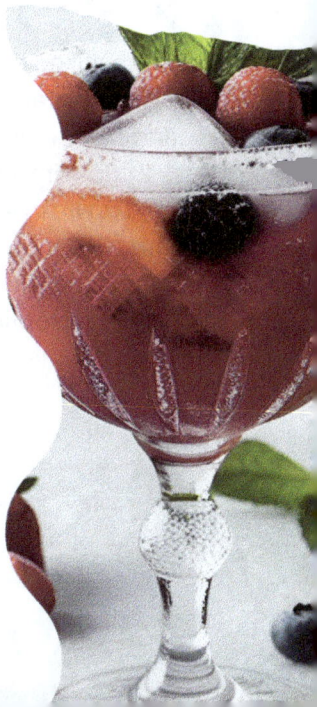

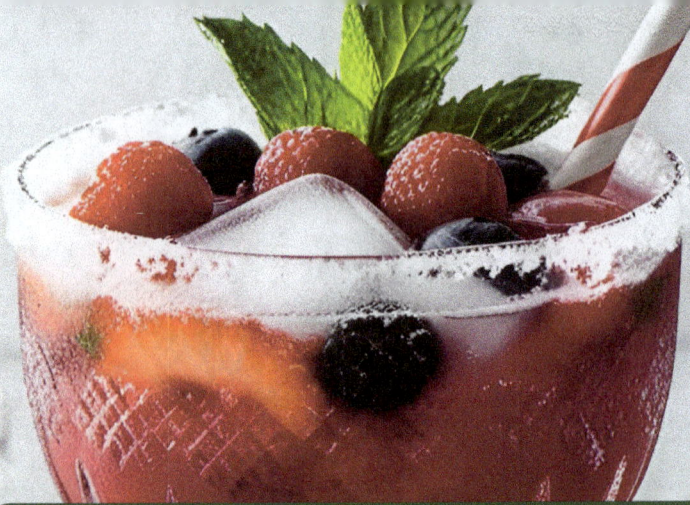

Winter Berry Punch

Berrylicious and bursting with color—your winter table's new favorite punch.

Serving Size	Serving Time
4 people	10 min.

Ingredients

- 1 cup mixed berry puree (from a blend of strawberries, raspberries, and blueberries)
- 1/2 cup mint syrup
- 1/2 cup fresh lemon juice (from about 2 lemons)
- 3 cups soda water
- Ice cubes (optional)
- Fresh mint leaves and berries for garnish

Procedure

1. In a blender, puree the mixed berries until smooth. Strain through a fine mesh sieve to remove seeds if desired.
2. In a pitcher, combine the berry puree, mint syrup, and lemon juice. Stir well.
3. Add the soda water and stir gently.
4. Fill four glasses with ice (if using) and pour the mocktail mixture into the glasses.
5. Garnish with fresh mint leaves and berries before serving.

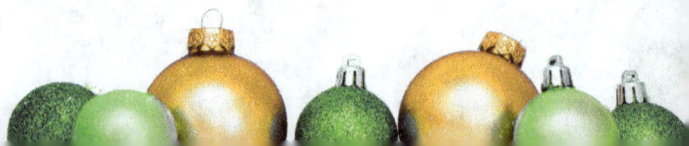

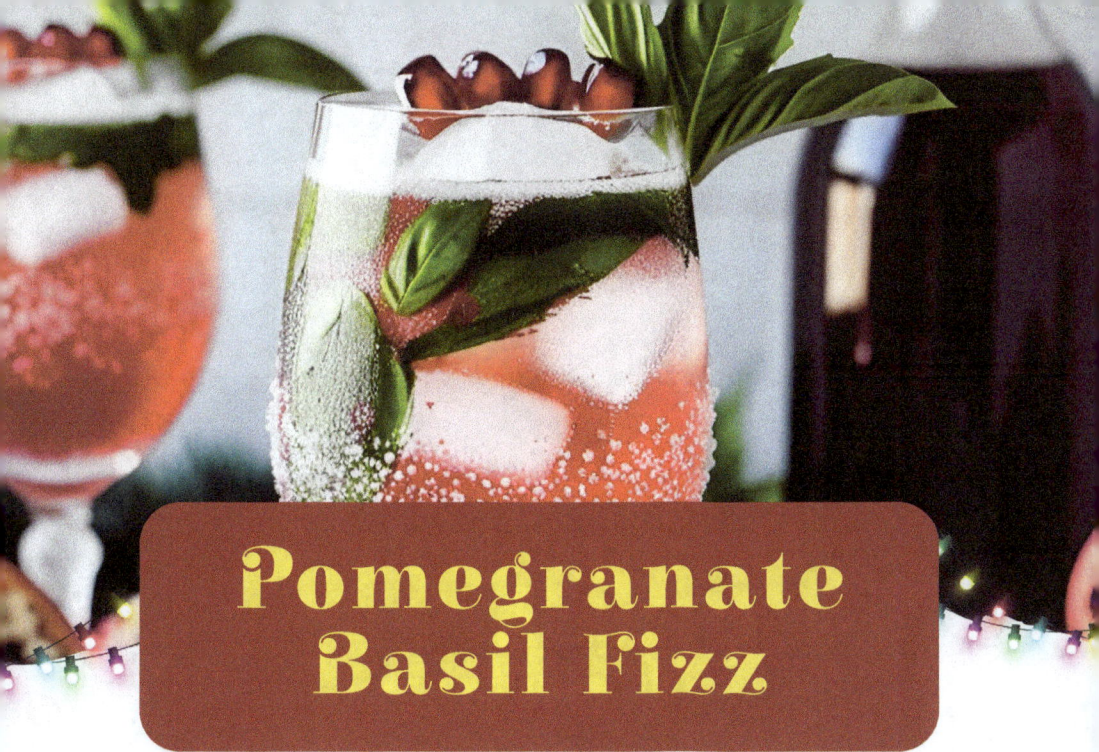

Pomegranate Basil Fizz

A garden-fresh twist with ruby red sparkle—unexpected and irresistible.

Serving Size	Serving Time
4 people	10 min.

Ingredients

- 2 cups fresh pomegranate juice (from about 2 large pomegranates)
- 1/2 cup basil syrup
- 3 cups club soda
- Ice cubes (optional)
- Fresh basil leaves and pomegranate seeds for garnish

Procedure

1. In a pitcher, combine the pomegranate juice and basil syrup. Stir well.
2. Add the club soda and stir gently.
3. Fill four glasses with ice (if using) and pour the mocktail mixture into the glasses.
4. Garnish with fresh basil leaves and pomegranate seeds before serving.

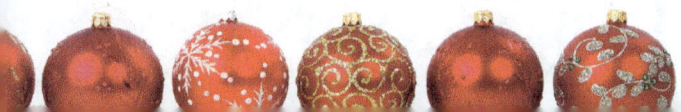

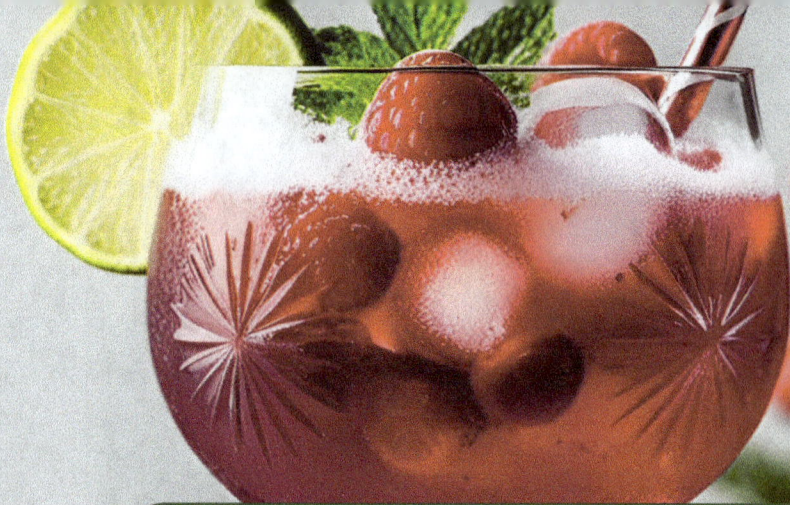

Raspberry & Cranberry Cooler

A tangy duo that dances on your tongue—berry bliss with a citrus kiss.

Serving Size	Serving Time
4 people	10 min.

Ingredients

- 1 cup fresh raspberry juice (from about 2 cups of raspberries, pureed and strained)
- 1 cup fresh cranberry juice
- 1/2 cup fresh lime juice (from about 4 limes)
- 3 cups soda water
- Ice cubes (optional)
- Fresh raspberries and lime wedges for garnish

Procedure

1. In a pitcher, combine the raspberry juice, cranberry juice, and lime juice. Stir well.
2. Add the soda water and stir gently.
3. Fill four glasses with ice (if using) and pour the mocktail mixture into the glasses.
4. Garnish with fresh raspberries and lime wedges before serving.

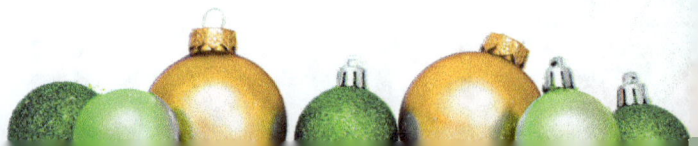

Blackberry Ginger Ale

Juicy blackberries meet zesty ginger for a fizzy holiday treat.

Serving Size	Serving Time
4 people	10 min.

Ingredients

- 2 cups fresh blackberry puree (from about 2 cups of blackberries, pureed and strained)
- 1/2 cup ginger syrup
- 3 cups soda water
- Ice cubes (optional)
- Fresh blackberries and ginger slices for garnish

Procedure

1. In a blender, puree the blackberries until smooth. Strain the mixture through a fine mesh sieve to remove seeds if desired.
2. In a pitcher, combine the blackberry puree and ginger syrup. Stir well.
3. Add the soda water and stir gently.
4. Fill four glasses with ice (if using) and pour the mocktail mixture into the glasses.
5. Garnish with fresh blackberries and ginger slices before serving.

Blueberry Spice Mocktail

Warm spice and cool blueberries mingle in this winter wonder.

Serving Size	Serving Time
4 people	10 min.

Ingredients

- 2 cups fresh blueberry juice (from about 3 cups of blueberries, pureed and strained)
- 1/2 cup cinnamon syrup
- 3 cups soda water
- Ice cubes (optional)
- Fresh blueberries and cinnamon sticks for garnish

Procedure

1. In a pitcher, combine the blueberry juice and cinnamon syrup. Stir well.
2. Add the soda water and stir gently.
3. Fill four glasses with ice (if using) and pour the mocktail mixture into the glasses.
4. Garnish with fresh blueberries and a cinnamon stick before serving.

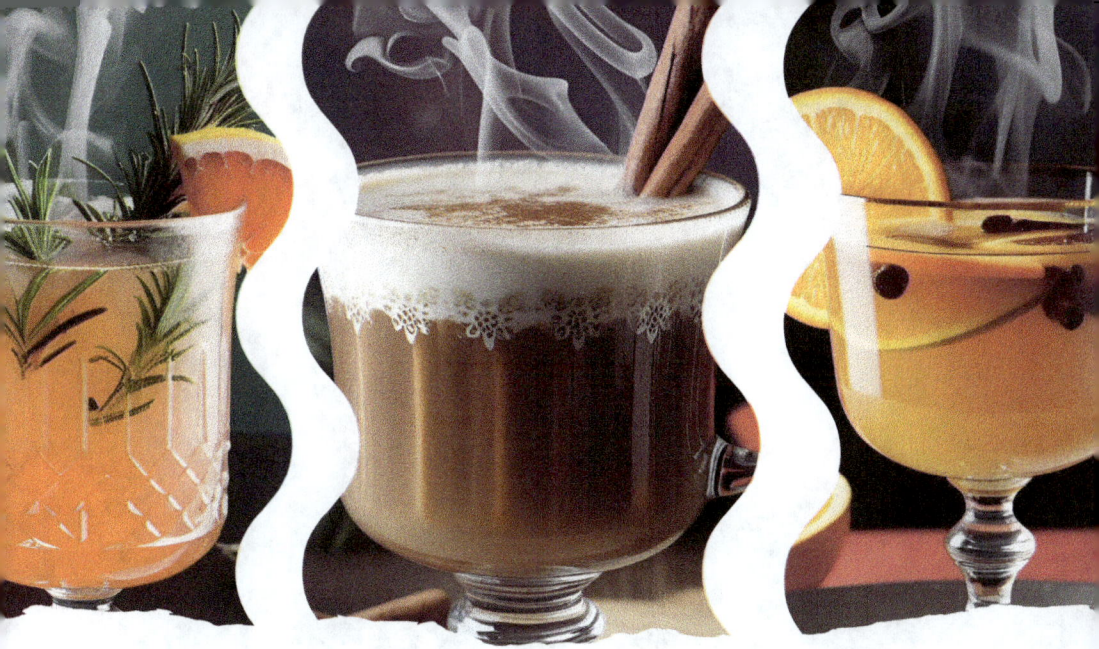

WARM SPICE AND HERBAL MOCKTAILS

These warm spice and herbal mocktails are perfect for cozying up during the winter season, bringing warmth and festive flavors to your gatherings.

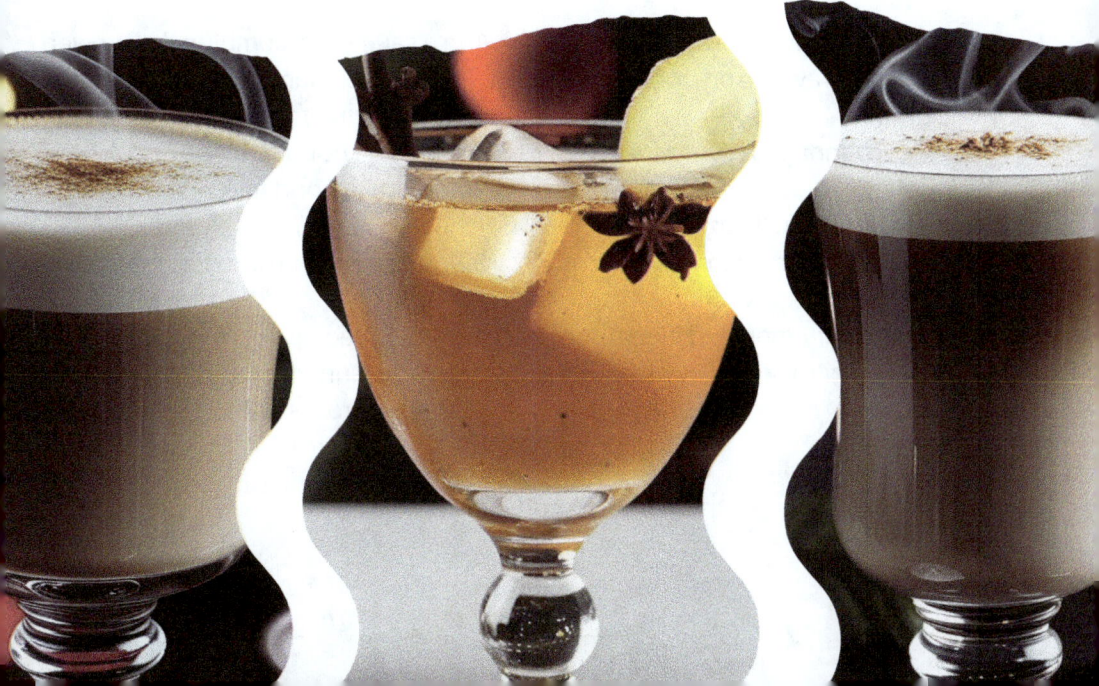

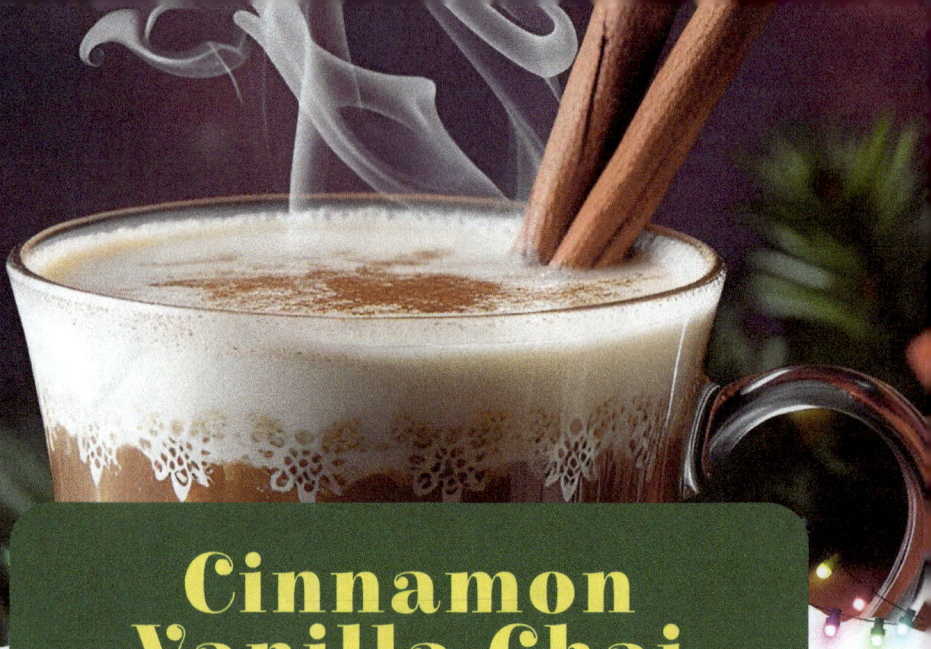

Cinnamon Vanilla Chai

Aromatic, spicy, and creamy—a fireside favorite in every cozy cup.

Serving Size	Serving Time
4 people	10 min.

Ingredients

- 2 cups freshly brewed chai tea (strongly brewed and cooled slightly)
- 1/2 cup cinnamon syrup (recipe below)
- 1 teaspoon vanilla extract
- 1 cup almond milk (or any milk of your choice)
- Ground cinnamon and cinnamon sticks for garnish

Procedure

1. In a saucepan, combine the brewed chai tea, cinnamon syrup, and vanilla extract. Warm over medium heat until hot but not boiling.
2. Add the almond milk and stir until heated through.
3. Pour the mixture into four heatproof mugs.
4. Garnish each mug with a sprinkle of ground cinnamon and a cinnamon stick before serving.

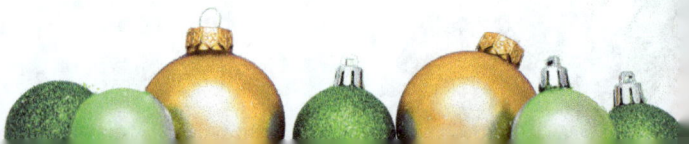

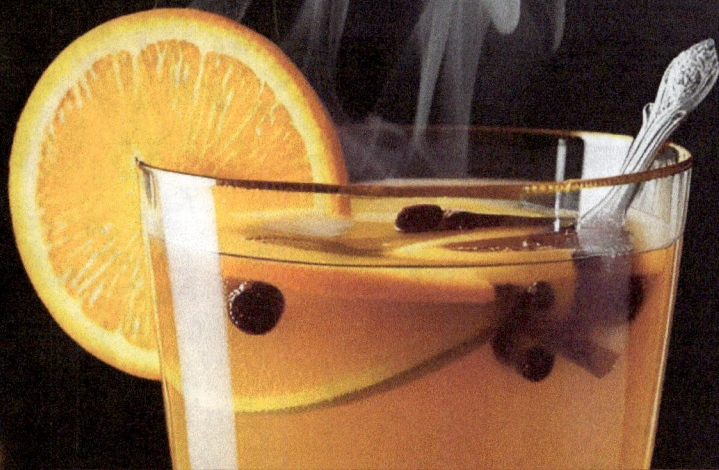

Spiced Orange Punch

Citrus and spice come together for a punch that's pure seasonal joy.

Serving Size	Serving Time
4 people	10 min.

Ingredients

- 2 cups fresh orange juice (from about 4-5 oranges)
- 1/2 cup spiced syrup (recipe below)
- 2 cups warm water
- Orange slices and star anise for garnish

Procedure

1. In a saucepan, combine the fresh orange juice, spiced syrup, and warm water. Heat over medium-low heat until warm (do not boil).
2. Pour the mixture into four heatproof mugs.
3. Garnish each mug with an orange slice and a star anise before serving.

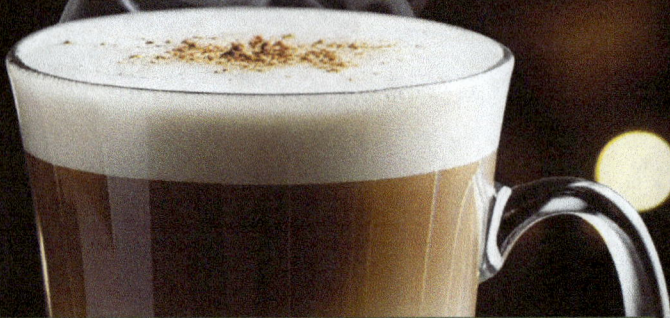

Nutmeg Maple Latte

Rich coffee, smooth maple, and warm nutmeg—your morning just got festive.

Serving Size	Serving Time
4 people	10 min.

Ingredients

- 2 cups freshly brewed coffee (hot)
- 1/2 cup maple syrup
- 1/2 teaspoon freshly grated nutmeg
- 2 cups almond milk (or any milk of your choice)
- Ground nutmeg for garnish

Procedure

1. In a saucepan, combine the brewed coffee, maple syrup, and freshly grated nutmeg. Heat over medium heat until hot.
2. Add the almond milk and stir until heated through.
3. Pour the mixture into four heatproof mugs.
4. Garnish each mug with a sprinkle of ground nutmeg before serving.

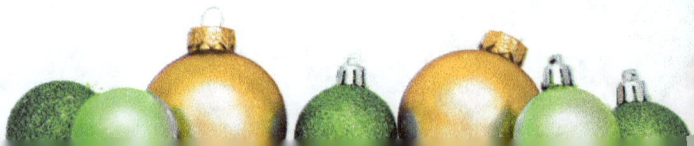

Rosemary Citrus Warm-Up

Herbal and invigorating with a citrus kick—like a snowy forest walk in a mug.

Serving Size	Serving Time
4 people	10 min.

Ingredients

- 2 cups fresh grapefruit juice (from about 2 large grapefruits)
- 1/2 cup rosemary syrup (recipe below)
- 2 cups warm water
- Fresh rosemary sprigs and grapefruit slices for garnish

Procedure

1. In a saucepan, combine the grapefruit juice, rosemary syrup, and warm water. Heat over medium-low heat until warm (do not boil).
2. Pour the mixture into four heatproof mugs.
3. Garnish each mug with a fresh rosemary sprig and a grapefruit slice before serving.

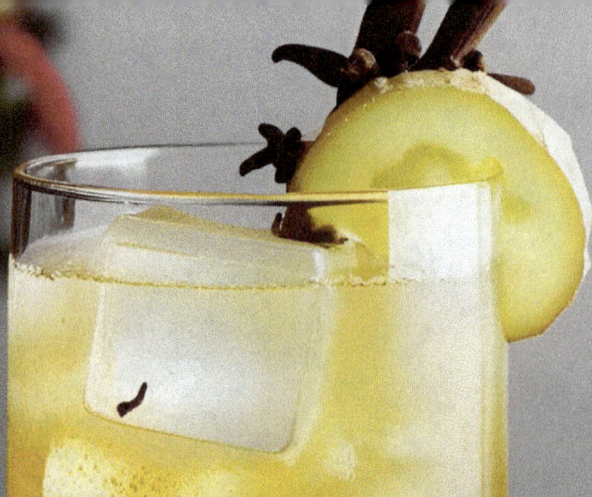

Clove & Ginger Tonic

A bold and bracing blend of clove and ginger—pep-in-your-step included.

Serving Size	Serving Time
4 people	10 min.

Ingredients

- 1 cup fresh ginger juice (from about 4 inches of ginger root, grated and juiced)
- 1/2 cup clove syrup (recipe below)
- 2 cups tonic water
- Ice cubes (optional)
- Fresh ginger slices and whole cloves for garnish

Procedure

1. In a pitcher, combine the ginger juice and clove syrup. Stir well.
2. Add the tonic water and stir gently.
3. Fill four glasses with ice (if using) and pour the mocktail mixture into the glasses.
4. Garnish each glass with fresh ginger slices and a few whole cloves before serving.

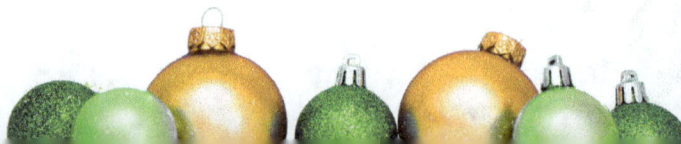

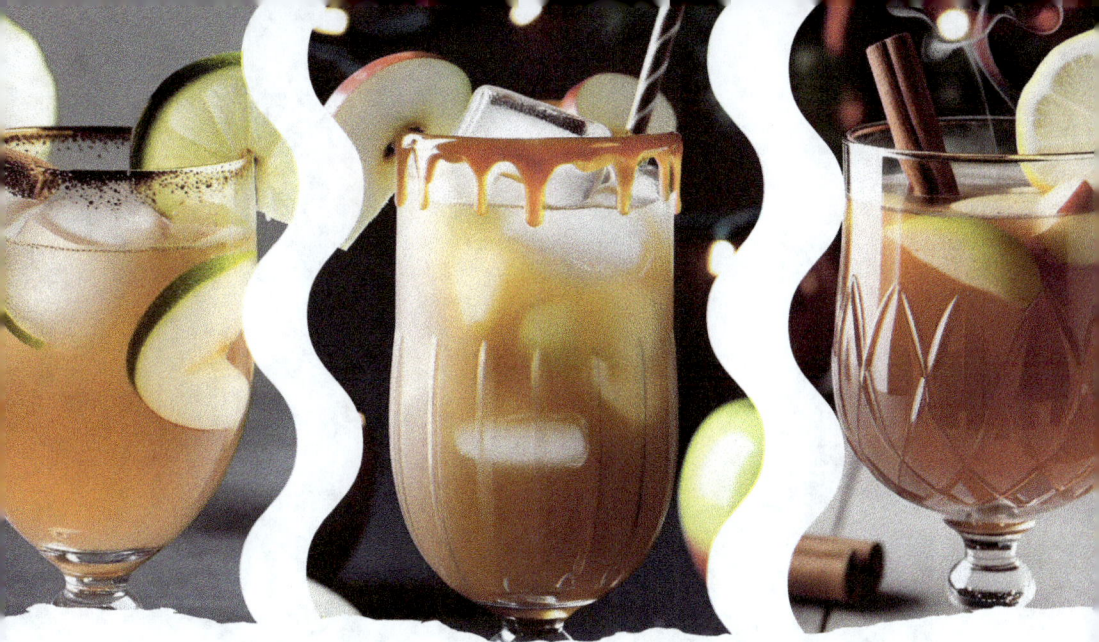

PEAR & APPLE CREATIONS

These pear and apple mocktails bring warm, comforting flavors perfect for the holiday season.

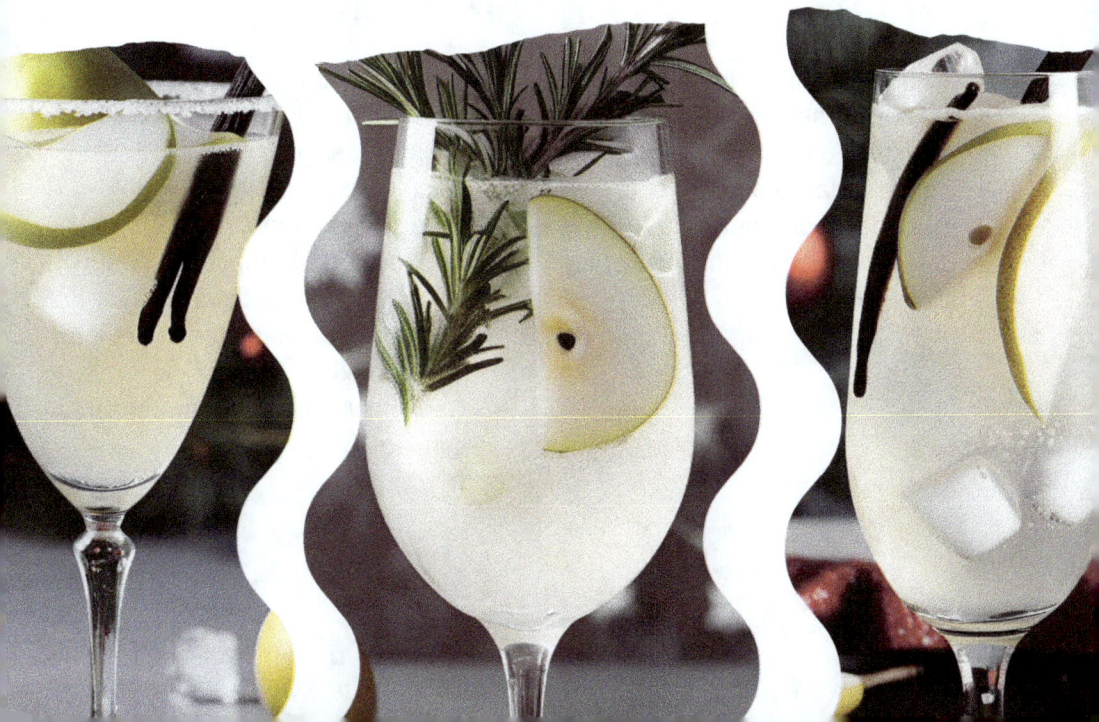

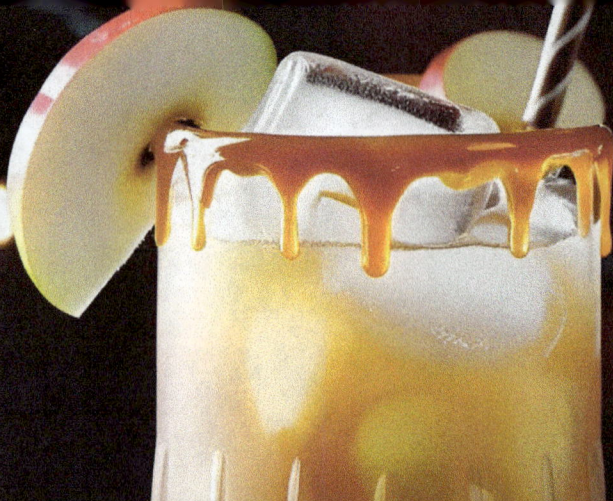

Caramel Apple Cooler

Sweet, fizzy, and nostalgic—like biting into a caramel-dipped apple.

Serving Size	Serving Time
4 people	10 min.

Ingredients

- 2 cups fresh apple juice
- 1/2 cup caramel syrup (recipe below)
- 3 cups soda water
- Ice cubes (optional)
- Caramel sauce for rim and apple slices for garnish

Procedure

1. To prepare the glasses, dip the rims in caramel sauce, then coat with sugar if desired.
2. In a pitcher, combine the apple juice and caramel syrup. Stir well.
3. Add the soda water and stir gently.
4. Fill four glasses with ice (if using) and pour the mocktail mixture into the glasses.
5. Garnish with apple slices before serving.

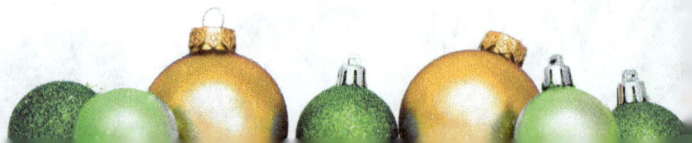

Pear & Vanilla Fizz

Smooth, mellow, and softly sweet—a pear-fect winter refresher.

Serving Size	Serving Time
4 people	10 min.

Ingredients

- 2 cups fresh pear juice (from about 4 ripe pears, pureed and strained)
- 1/2 cup vanilla syrup (recipe below)
- 3 cups soda water
- Ice cubes (optional)
- Fresh pear slices and vanilla bean for garnish

Procedure

1. In a pitcher, combine the fresh pear juice and vanilla syrup. Stir well.
2. Add the soda water and stir gently.
3. Fill four glasses with ice (if using) and pour the mocktail mixture into the glasses.
4. Garnish with fresh pear slices and a vanilla bean before serving.

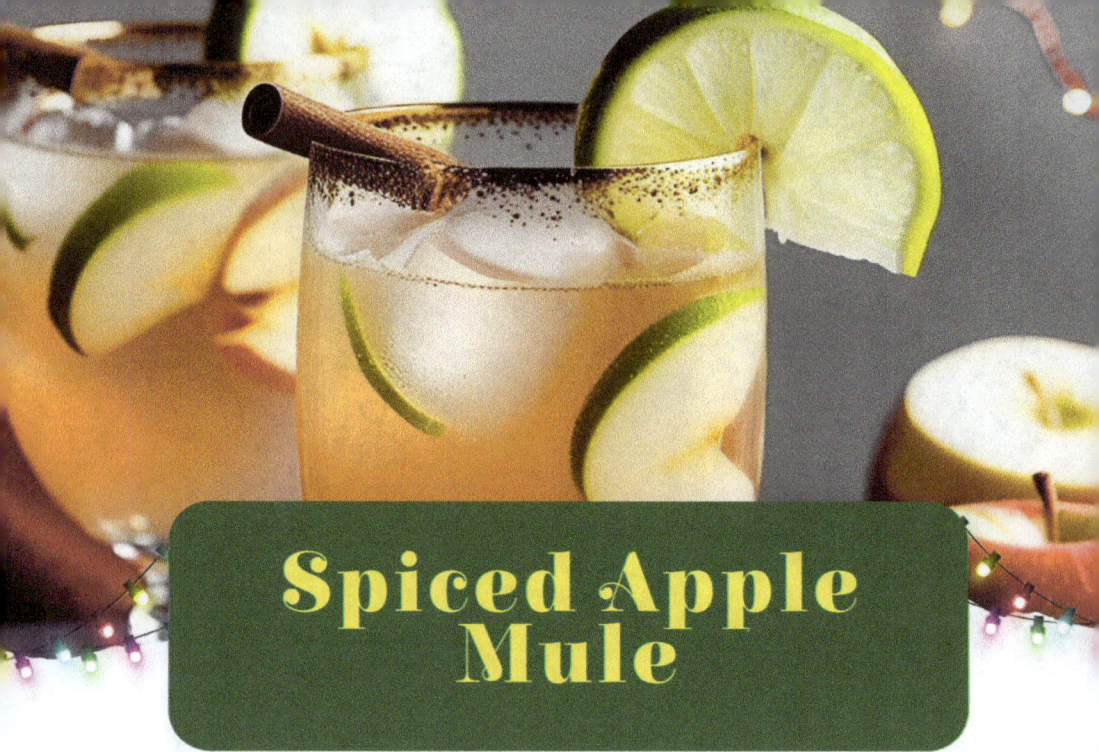

Spiced Apple Mule

Tart apple and bold ginger with a festive lime twist—holiday-ready and oh-so-sippable.

Serving Size	Serving Time
4 people	10 min.

Ingredients

- 2 cups fresh apple juice
- 1/2 cup ginger syrup (recipe below)
- 1/4 cup fresh lime juice (from about 2 limes)
- 3 cups soda water
- Ice cubes
- Fresh lime wedges and apple slices for garnish

Procedure

1. In a pitcher, combine the apple juice, ginger syrup, and lime juice. Stir well.
2. Add the soda water and stir gently.
3. Fill four copper mugs or glasses with ice and pour the mocktail mixture into the glasses.
4. Garnish with lime wedges and apple slices before serving.

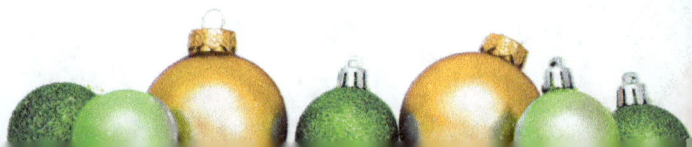

Warm Apple Cinnamon Toddy

Toasty and fragrant, like your favorite cinnamon-apple candle in liquid form.

Serving Size	Serving Time
4 people	10 min.

Ingredients

- 3 cups fresh apple cider
- 1/2 cup cinnamon infusion (recipe below)
- 1 tablespoon fresh lemon juice
- Cinnamon sticks and lemon slices for garnish

Procedure

1. In a saucepan, combine the apple cider, cinnamon infusion, and lemon juice. Heat over medium-low heat until warm (do not boil).
2. Pour the mixture into four heatproof mugs.
3. Garnish each mug with a cinnamon stick and a lemon slice before serving.

Pear & Rosemary Sparkler

Subtle and sophisticated with herbal elegance—a showstopper for winter nights.

Serving Size	Serving Time
4 people	10 min.

Ingredients

- 2 cups fresh pear juice (from about 4 ripe pears, pureed and strained)
- 1/2 cup rosemary syrup (recipe below)
- 3 cups tonic water
- Ice cubes (optional)
- Fresh rosemary sprigs and pear slices for garnish

Procedure

1. In a pitcher, combine the pear juice and rosemary syrup. Stir well.
2. Add the tonic water and stir gently.
3. Fill four glasses with ice (if using) and pour the mocktail mixture into the glasses.
4. Garnish with fresh rosemary sprigs and pear slices before serving.

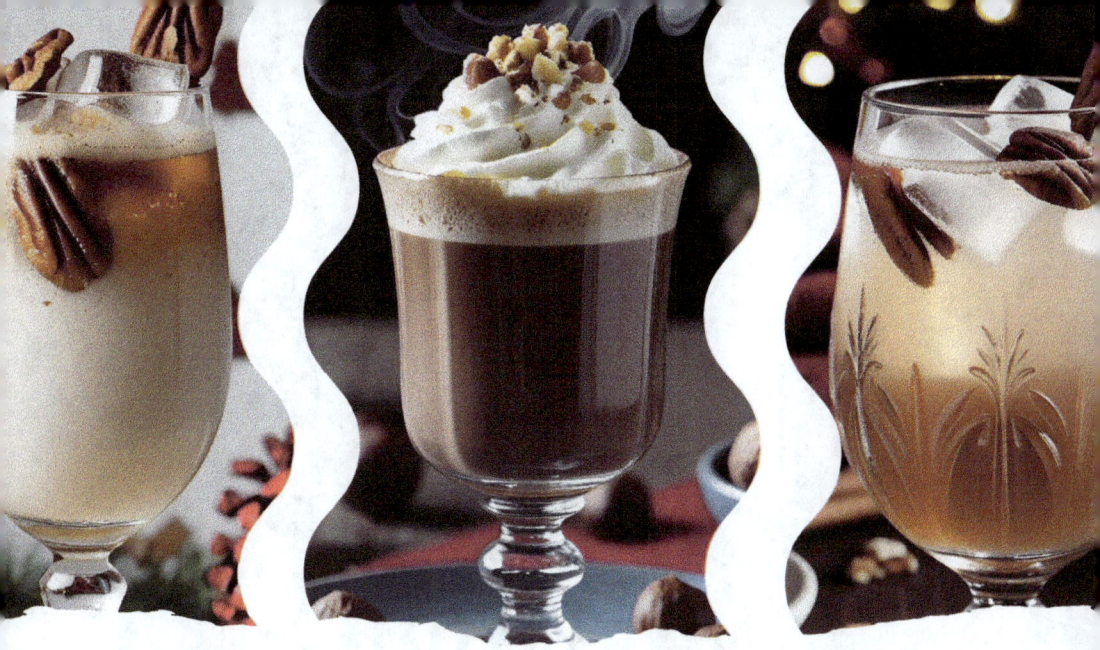

NUTTY AND CREAMY MOCKTAILS

These nutty and creamy mocktails provide comforting and indulgent flavors perfect for holiday gatherings or cozy nights in.

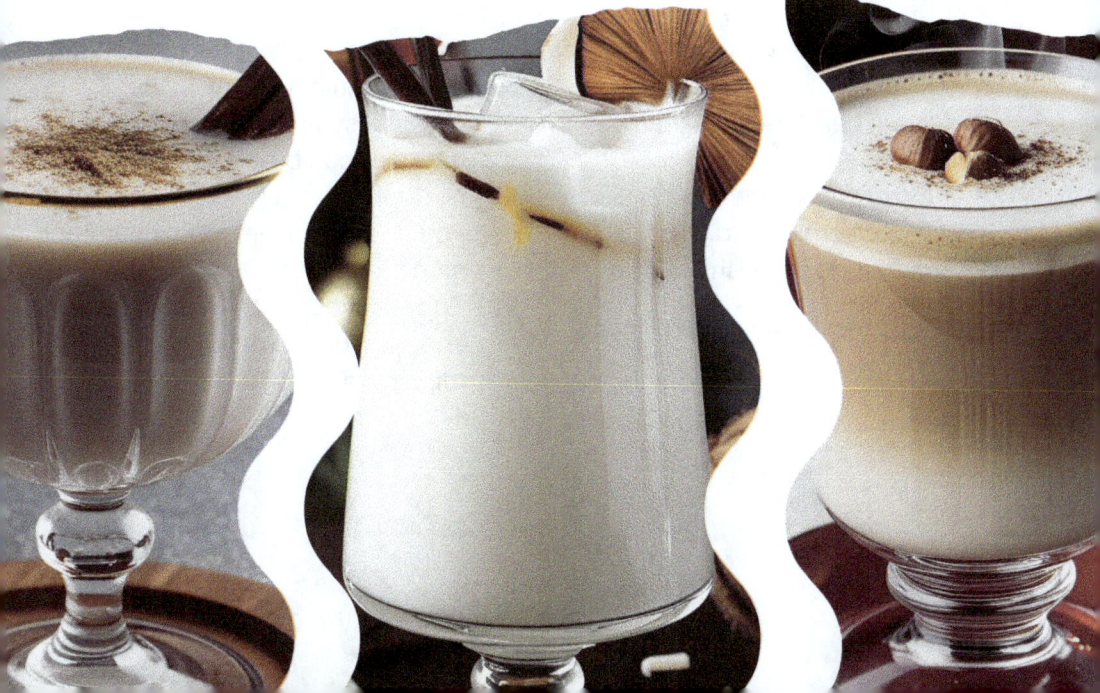

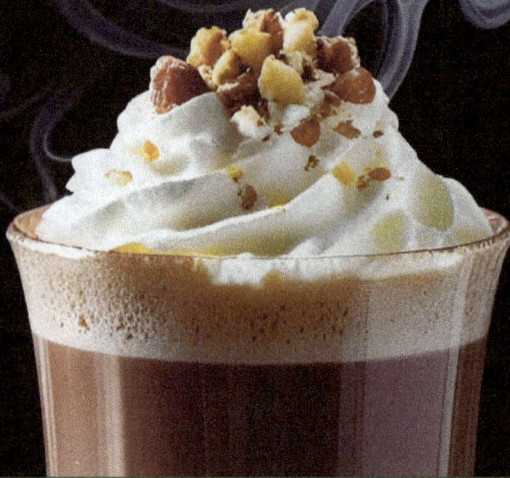

Toasted Hazelnut Chocolate

Dreamy hazelnut and rich cocoa—like Nutella in a mug!

Serving Size	Serving Time
4 people	10 min.

Ingredients

- 2 cups almond milk (or any milk of your choice)
- 1/2 cup hazelnut syrup (recipe below)
- 1/2 cup cocoa powder
- Whipped cream and crushed hazelnuts for garnish

Procedure

1. In a saucepan, heat the almond milk over medium heat. Stir in the hazelnut syrup and cocoa powder until well combined and warm (do not boil).
2. Pour the mixture into four heatproof mugs.
3. Top each mug with whipped cream and sprinkle crushed hazelnuts on top before serving.

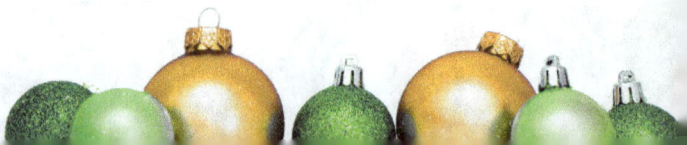

Maple Pecan Fizz

Creamy pecan milk and maple bubbles—an indulgent twist on tradition.

Serving Size	Serving Time
4 people	10 min.

Ingredients

- 2 cups fresh pecan milk (recipe below)
- 1/2 cup maple syrup
- 3 cups soda water
- Dash of ground cinnamon
- Ice cubes (optional)
- Crushed pecans for garnish

Procedure

1. In a pitcher, combine the pecan milk and maple syrup. Stir well.
2. Add the soda water and stir gently.
3. Fill four glasses with ice (if using) and pour the mocktail mixture into the glasses.
4. Sprinkle with a dash of ground cinnamon and crushed pecans before serving.

Almond Spice Delight

Soft, nutty, and sweet with a whisper of warming spice.

Serving Size	Serving Time
4 people	10 min.

Ingredients

- 2 cups almond milk
- 1/2 cup cinnamon syrup (recipe below)
- 1 teaspoon vanilla extract
- Ground nutmeg for garnish

Procedure

1. In a saucepan, heat the almond milk over medium heat. Stir in the cinnamon syrup and vanilla extract until well combined and warm.
2. Pour the mixture into four heatproof mugs.
3. Sprinkle each mug with ground nutmeg before serving.

Coconut Cream Punch

Tropical flair meets wintry warmth—pure creamy joy.

Serving Size	Serving Time
4 people	10 min.

Ingredients

- 2 cups coconut milk (full-fat for creaminess)
- 1/2 teaspoon vanilla extract
- 1/4 teaspoon ground nutmeg
- Ice cubes (optional)
- Coconut flakes for garnish

Procedure

1. In a pitcher, combine the coconut milk, vanilla extract, and ground nutmeg. Stir well.
2. If serving cold, fill four glasses with ice and pour the mixture into the glasses. If serving warm, heat the mixture in a saucepan over medium heat before pouring into heatproof mugs.
3. Garnish with coconut flakes before serving.

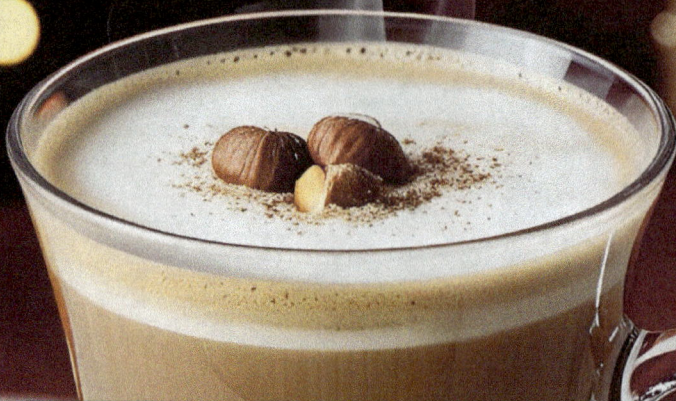

Warm Hazelnut Latte

Nutty, rich, and ultra-smooth—coffeehouse vibes from your own kitchen.

Serving Size	Serving Time
4 people	10 min.

Ingredients

- 2 cups brewed coffee (hot)
- 1/2 cup hazelnut syrup (recipe from Toasted Hazelnut Chocolate)
- 2 cups almond milk (frothed, if possible)
- Freshly grated nutmeg for garnish

Procedure

1. In a saucepan, combine the hot brewed coffee and hazelnut syrup. Stir until well mixed.
2. Divide the mixture into four heatproof mugs.
3. Top each mug with frothed almond milk.
4. Garnish with freshly grated nutmeg before serving.

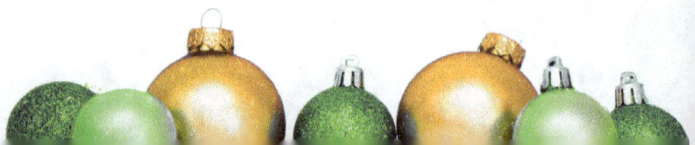

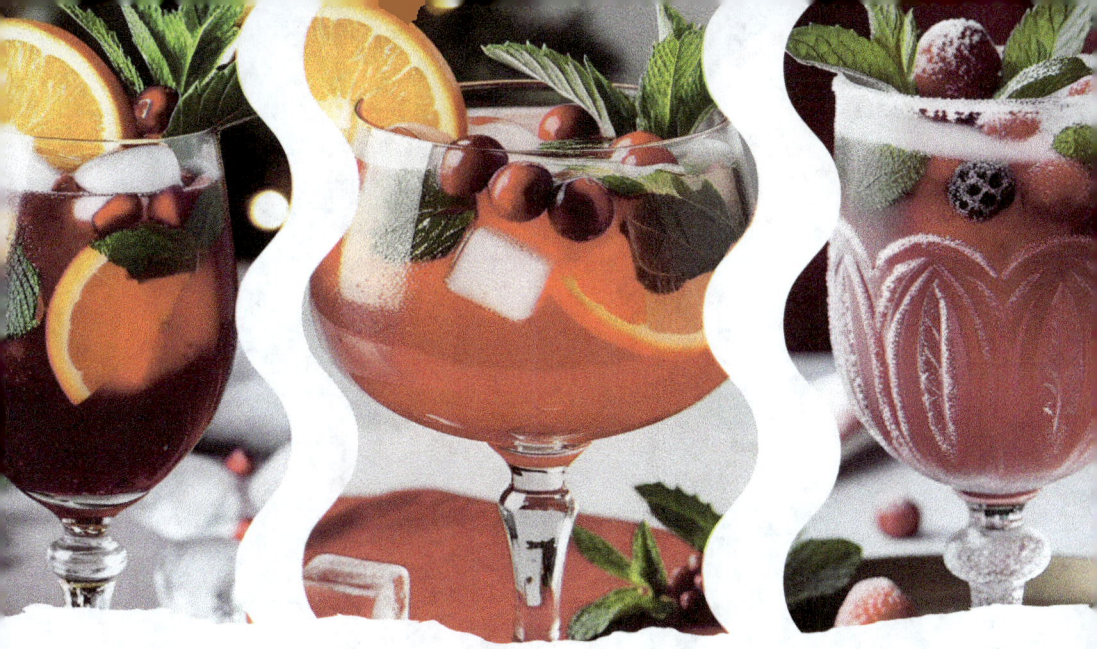

FESTIVE PUNCHES AND PARTY DRINKS

These syrups, cordials, and infusions are versatile and can be used to add depth and flavor to a variety of beverages and dishes.

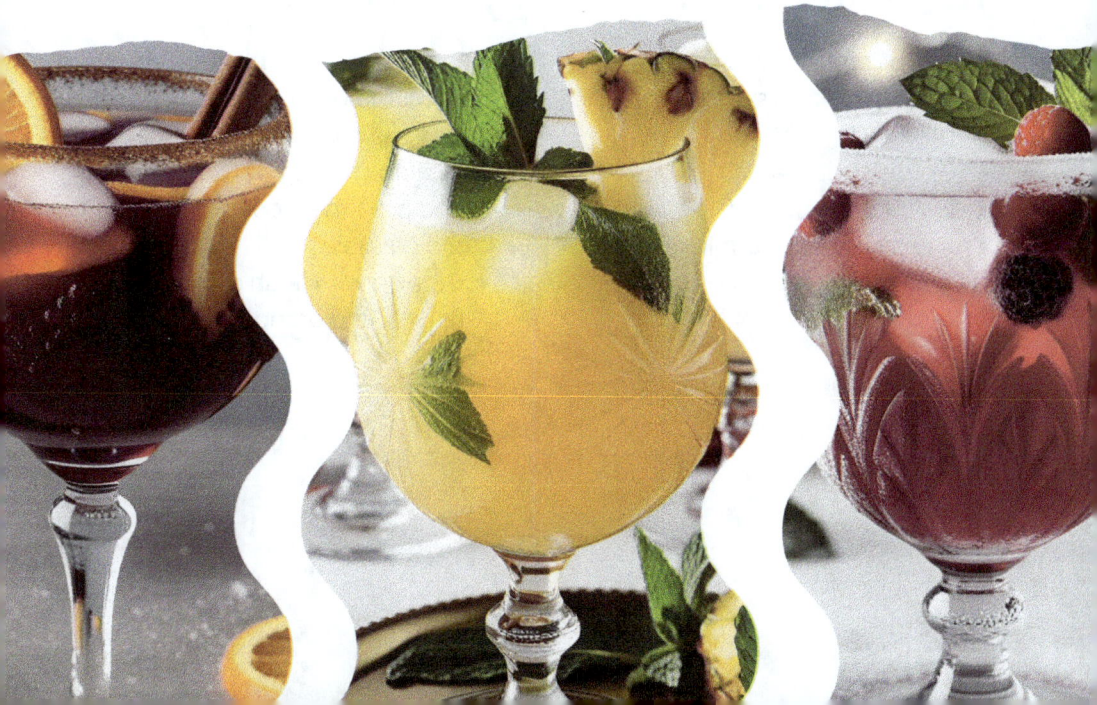

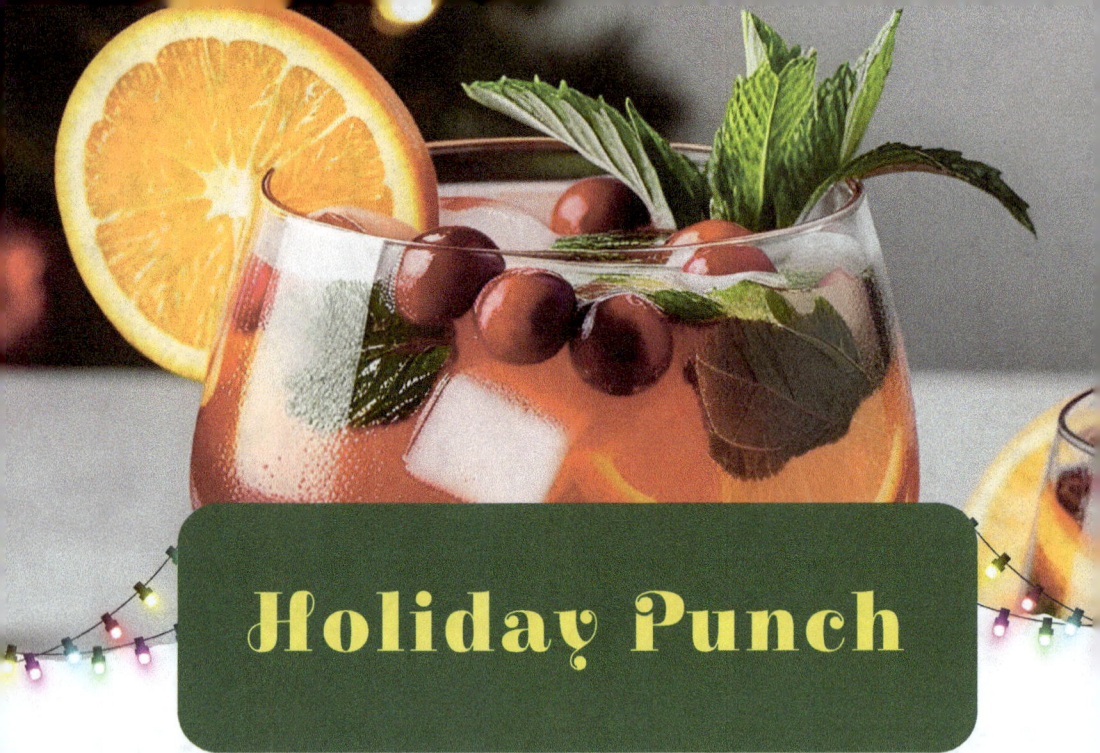

Holiday Punch

Bubbly, fruity, and filled with cheer—perfect for big bowls and happy hearts.

Serving Size	Serving Time
4 people	10 min.

Ingredients

- 2 cups cranberry juice
- 1/2 cup orange syrup (recipe below)
- 3 cups soda water
- Ice cubes (optional)
- Fresh cranberries, mint leaves, and orange slices for garnish

Procedure

1. In a pitcher, combine the cranberry juice and orange syrup. Stir well.
2. Add the soda water and stir gently.
3. Fill four glasses with ice (if using) and pour the mocktail mixture into the glasses.
4. Garnish with fresh cranberries, mint leaves, and orange slices before serving.

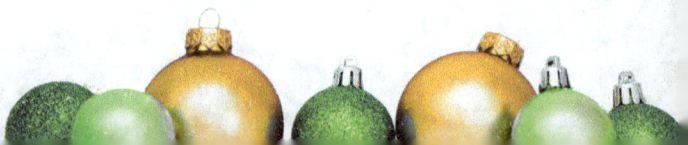

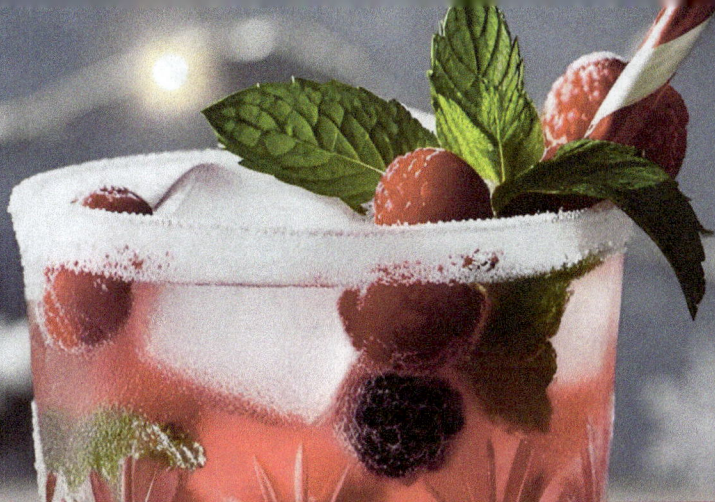

Frosted Berry Punch

Ice-cold and berry bright—like a snowflake party in a glass.

Serving Size	Serving Time
4 people	10 min.

Ingredients

- 2 cups mixed berry juice (from a blend of strawberries, raspberries, and blueberries, pureed and strained)
- 1/2 cup mint syrup (recipe below)
- 3 cups soda water
- Ice cubes (optional)
- Fresh berries and mint leaves for garnish

Procedure

1. In a pitcher, combine the mixed berry juice and mint syrup. Stir well.
2. Add the soda water and stir gently.
3. Fill four glasses with ice (if using) and pour the mocktail mixture into the glasses.
4. Garnish with fresh berries and mint leaves before serving.

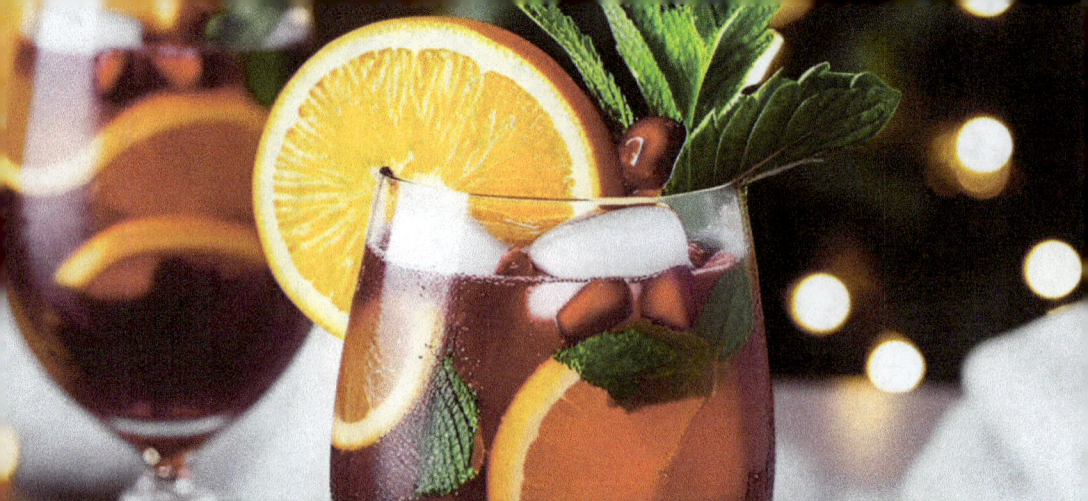

Sparkling Pomegranate Sangria

Deep red sparkle with citrus flair—your holiday table's sparkling star.

Serving Size	Serving Time
4 people	10 min.

Ingredients

- 2 cups fresh pomegranate juice (from about 2 large pomegranates)
- 1/2 cup fresh orange slices
- 3 cups soda water
- Ice cubes (optional)
- Fresh mint leaves and pomegranate seeds for garnish

Procedure

1. In a pitcher, combine the pomegranate juice and fresh orange slices. Stir gently to combine.
2. Add the soda water and stir lightly.
3. Fill four glasses with ice (if using) and pour the mocktail mixture into the glasses.
4. Garnish with fresh mint leaves and pomegranate seeds before serving.

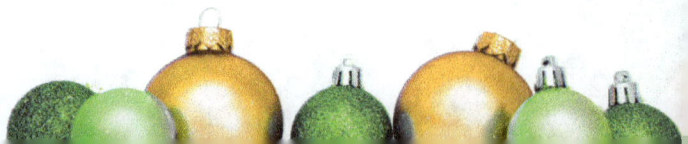

Winter Spice Mock Sangria

Cozy and complex, with grape, cinnamon, and zest—flavors that linger.

Serving Size	Serving Time
4 people	10 min.

Ingredients

- 2 cups fresh grape juice
- 1/2 teaspoon ground cinnamon
- Zest of 1 orange
- 3 cups soda water
- Ice cubes (optional)
- Fresh orange slices and cinnamon sticks for garnish

Procedure

1. In a pitcher, combine the pineapple juice and ginger syrup. Stir well.
2. Add the soda water and stir gently.
3. Fill four glasses with ice (if using) and pour the mocktail mixture into the glasses.
4. Garnish with fresh mint leaves and pineapple slices before serving.

Spiced Pineapple Punch

Juicy pineapple gets a warm, spicy twist—tropical meets twinkling.

Serving Size	Serving Time
4 people	10 min.

Ingredients

- 2 cups fresh pineapple juice
- 1/2 cup ginger syrup (recipe below)
- 3 cups soda water
- Ice cubes (optional)
- Fresh mint leaves and pineapple slices for garnish

Procedure

1. In a pitcher, combine the pineapple juice and ginger syrup. Stir well.
2. Add the soda water and stir gently.
3. Fill four glasses with ice (if using) and pour the mocktail mixture into the glasses.
4. Garnish with fresh mint leaves and pineapple slices before serving.

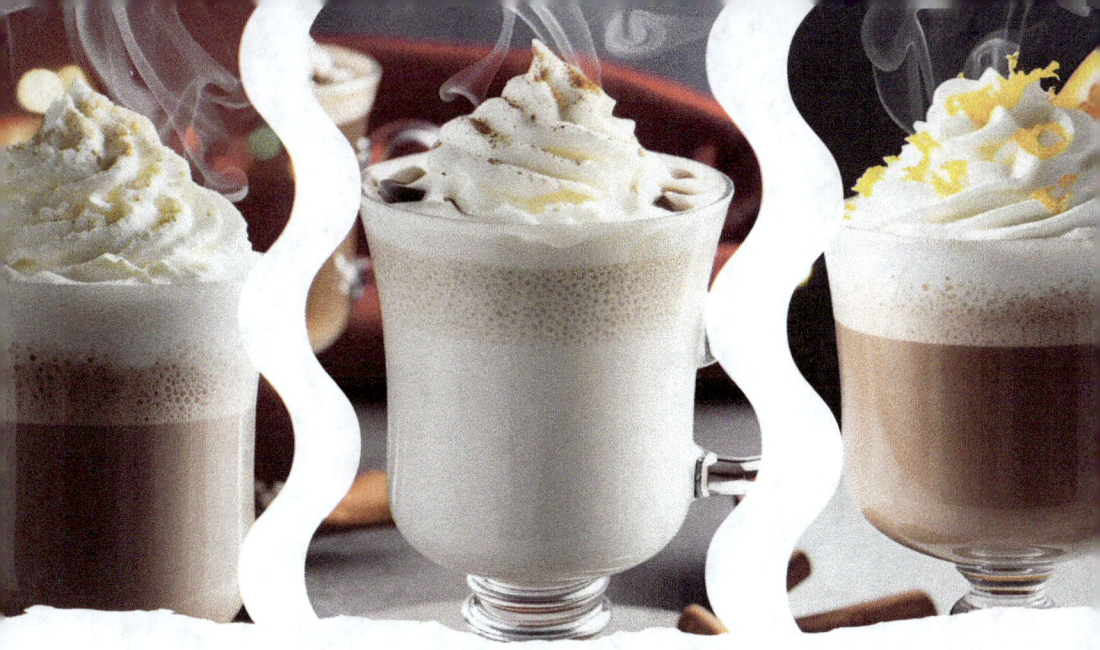

HOT CHOCOLATES & COZY DRINKS

These hot chocolates and cozy drinks are perfect for warming up on a cold winter's night, offering festive flavors to enjoy during the holiday season.

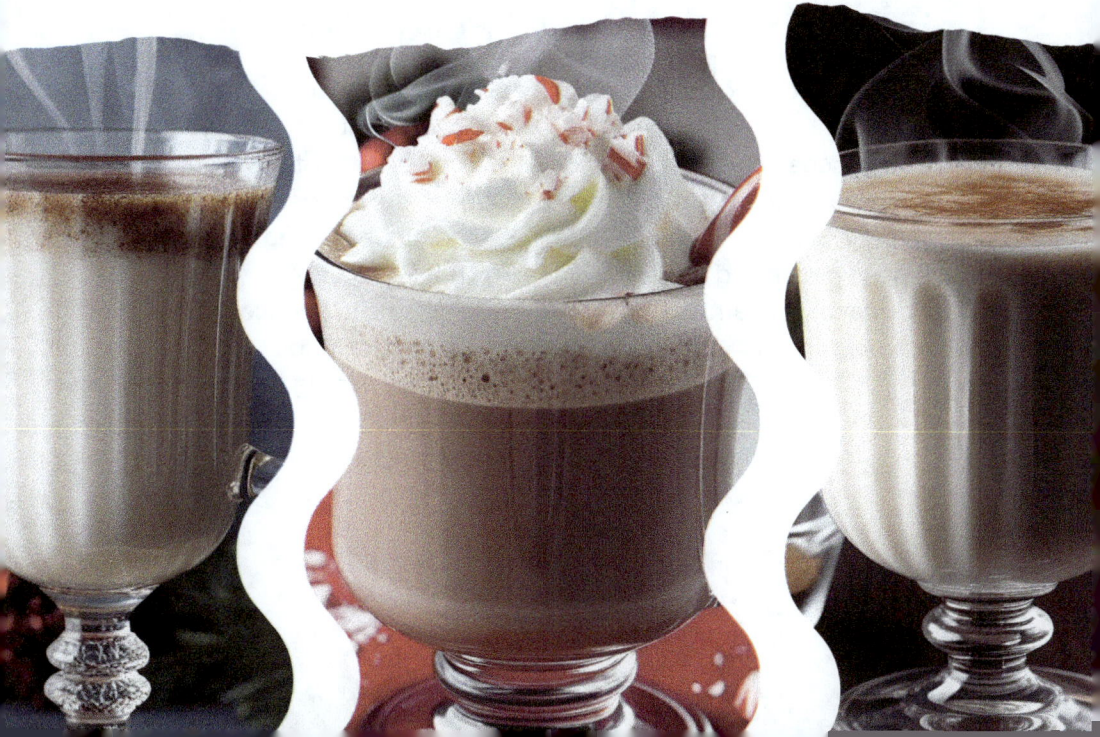

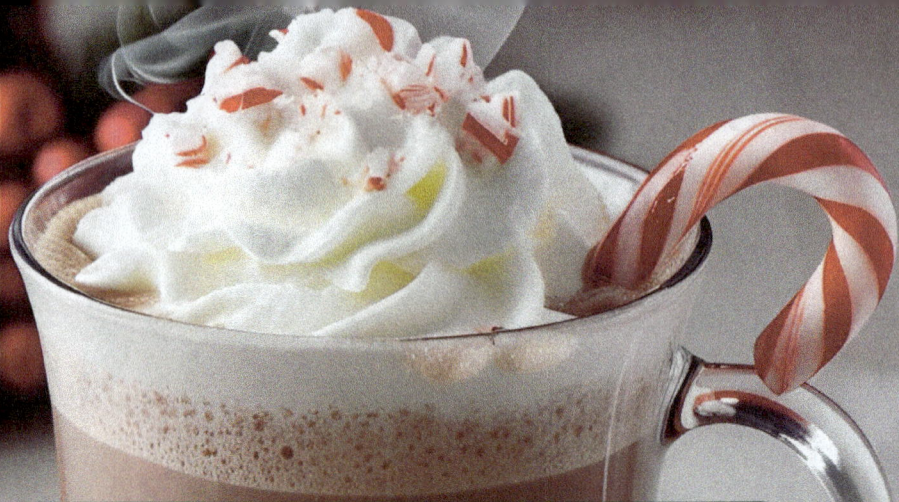

Peppermint Hot Chocolate

Cool mint, rich cocoa, and creamy warmth—it's the holidays in a mug.

Serving Size	Serving Time
4 people	10 min.

Ingredients

- 3 cups almond milk (or any milk of your choice)
- 1/2 cup cocoa powder
- 1/2 cup peppermint syrup (recipe below)
- Whipped cream and crushed candy canes for garnish

Procedure

1. In a saucepan, heat the almond milk over medium heat. Stir in the cocoa powder until it is well blended.
2. Add the peppermint syrup and continue heating until the mixture is hot (do not boil).
3. Pour the hot chocolate into four heatproof mugs.
4. Top each mug with whipped cream and crushed candy canes before serving.

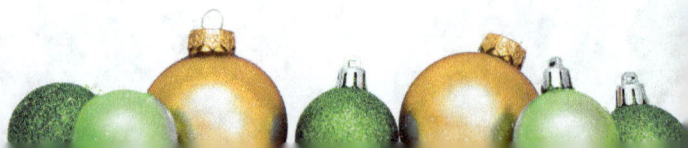

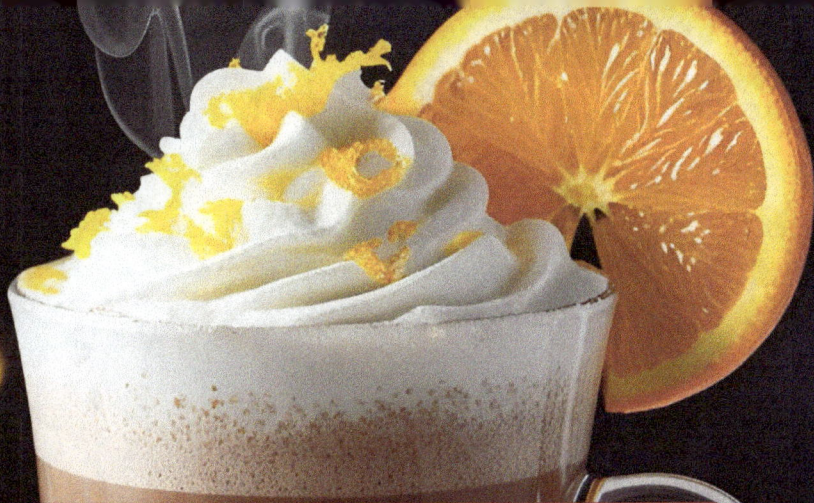

Cinnamon Orange Hot Cocoa

Bright citrus zest meets warming spice—unexpected and utterly divine.

Serving Size	Serving Time
4 people	10 min.

Ingredients

- 3 cups almond milk (or any milk of your choice)
- 1/2 cup cocoa powder
- 1/2 cup cinnamon syrup (recipe below)
- Zest of 1 orange
- Whipped cream and orange zest for garnish

Procedure

1. In a saucepan, heat the almond milk over medium heat. Stir in the cocoa powder and cinnamon syrup until well combined.
2. Add the orange zest and continue heating until the mixture is hot (do not boil).
3. Pour the hot cocoa into four heatproof mugs.
4. Top each mug with whipped cream and additional orange zest before serving.

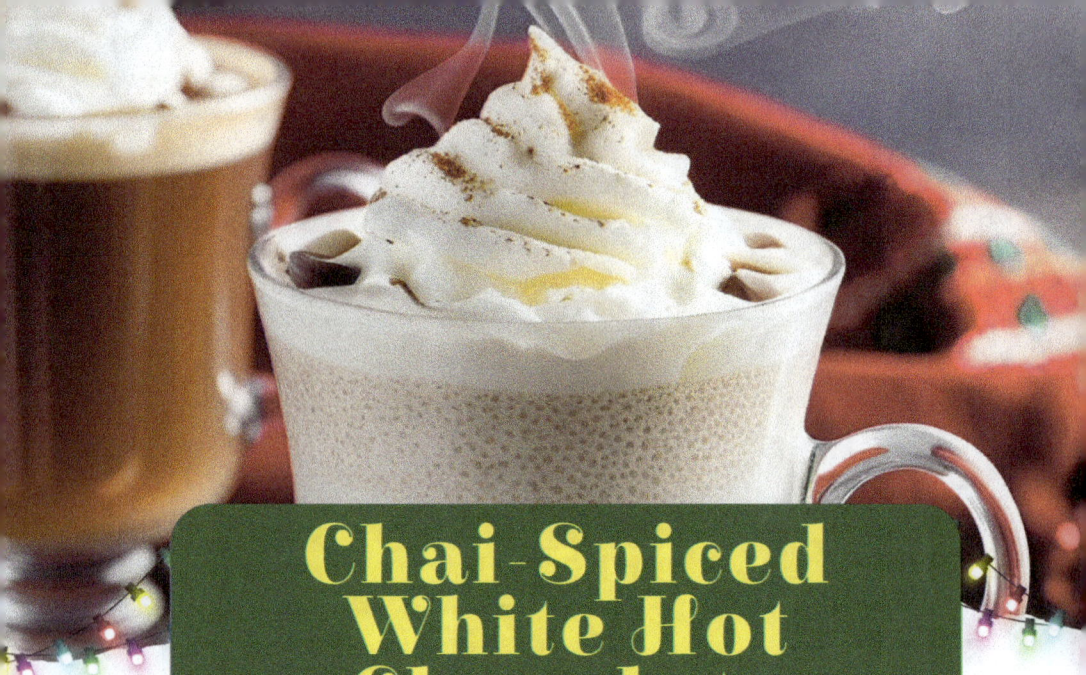

Chai-Spiced White Hot Chocolate

Sweet white chocolate and bold chai spice make this a winter white wonder.

Serving Size	Serving Time
4 people	10 min.

Ingredients

- 2 cups brewed chai tea (strongly brewed and cooled slightly)
- 3 cups almond milk (or any milk of your choice)
- 1/2 cup white chocolate chips
- Whipped cream and a sprinkle of cinnamon for garnish

Procedure

1. In a saucepan, combine the brewed chai tea and almond milk. Heat over medium heat until warm.
2. Add the white chocolate chips and stir until they are fully melted and the mixture is hot (do not boil).
3. Pour the white hot chocolate into four heatproof mugs.
4. Top each mug with whipped cream and a sprinkle of cinnamon before serving.

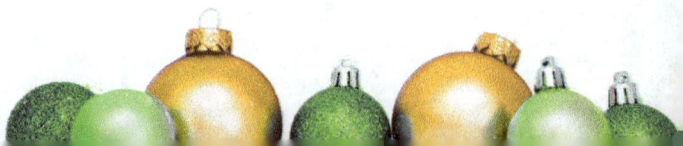

Hazelnut Cocoa Dream

Smooth, nutty, and velvety—like your dreamiest winter dessert.

Serving Size	Serving Time
4 people	10 min.

Ingredients

- 3 cups almond milk (or any milk of your choice)
- 1/2 cup cocoa powder
- 1/2 cup hazelnut syrup (recipe below)
- Whipped cream and grated nutmeg for garnish

Procedure

1. In a saucepan, heat the almond milk over medium heat. Stir in the cocoa powder until well blended.
2. Add the hazelnut syrup and continue heating until the mixture is hot (do not boil).
3. Pour the hot cocoa into four heatproof mugs.
4. Top each mug with whipped cream and a sprinkle of grated nutmeg before serving.

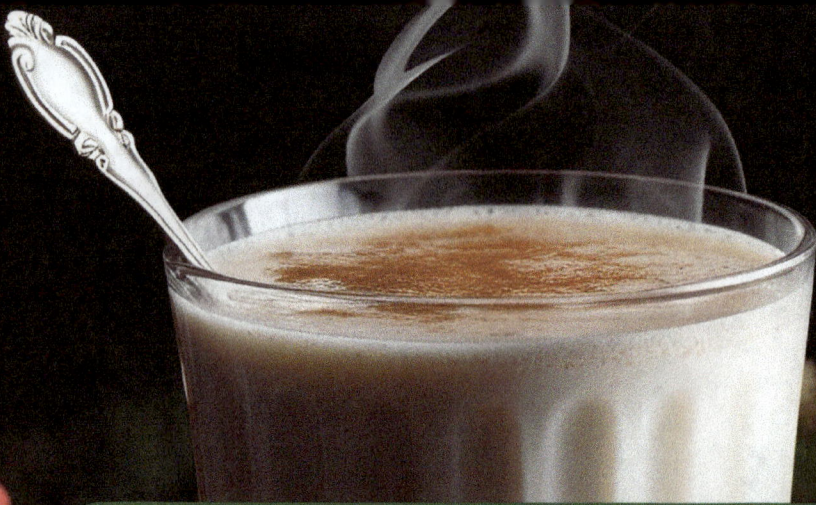

Spiced Vanilla Almond Milk

Comforting, creamy, and gently spiced—your new bedtime favorite.

Serving Size	Serving Time
4 people	10 min.

Ingredients

- 3 cups almond milk
- 1/2 cup cinnamon syrup (recipe above)
- 1 teaspoon vanilla extract
- Ground cinnamon for garnish

Procedure

1. In a saucepan, heat the almond milk over medium heat. Stir in the cinnamon syrup and vanilla extract until well combined and warm.
2. Pour the spiced almond milk into four heatproof mugs.
3. Sprinkle each mug with ground cinnamon before serving.

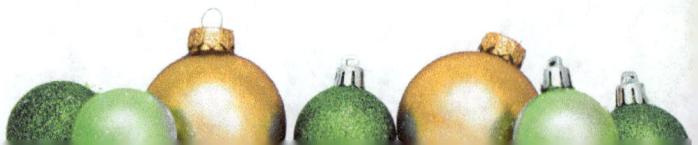

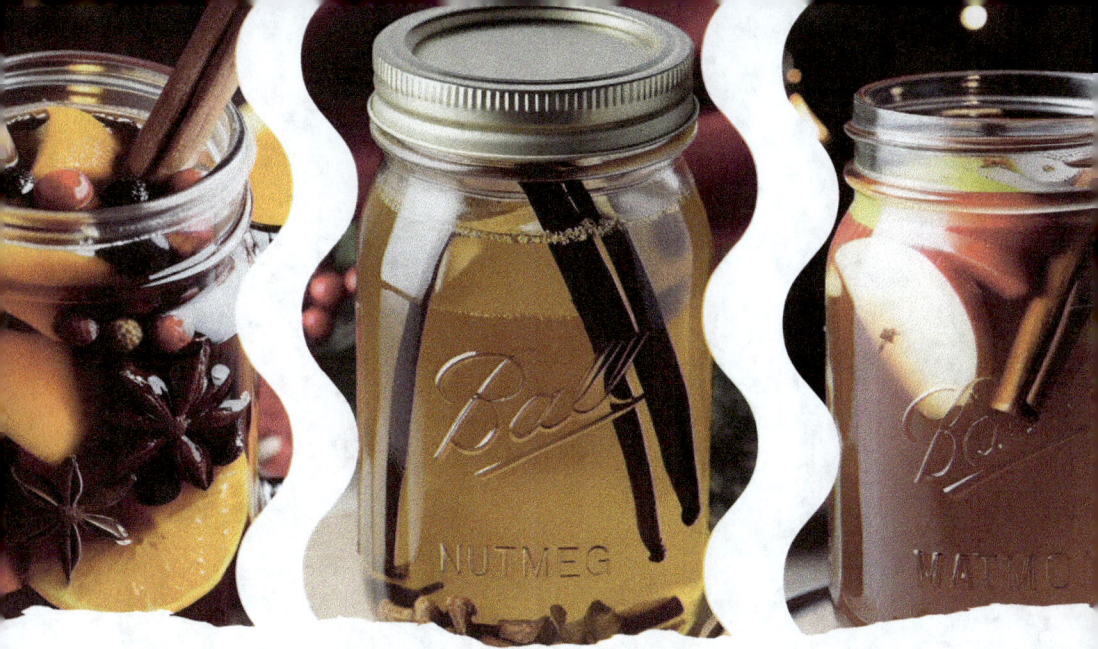

HOMEMADE SYRUPS, CORDIALS, AND INFUSIONS

These syrups, cordials, and infusions are versatile and perfect for adding festive flavors to holiday mocktails, cocktails, or desserts.

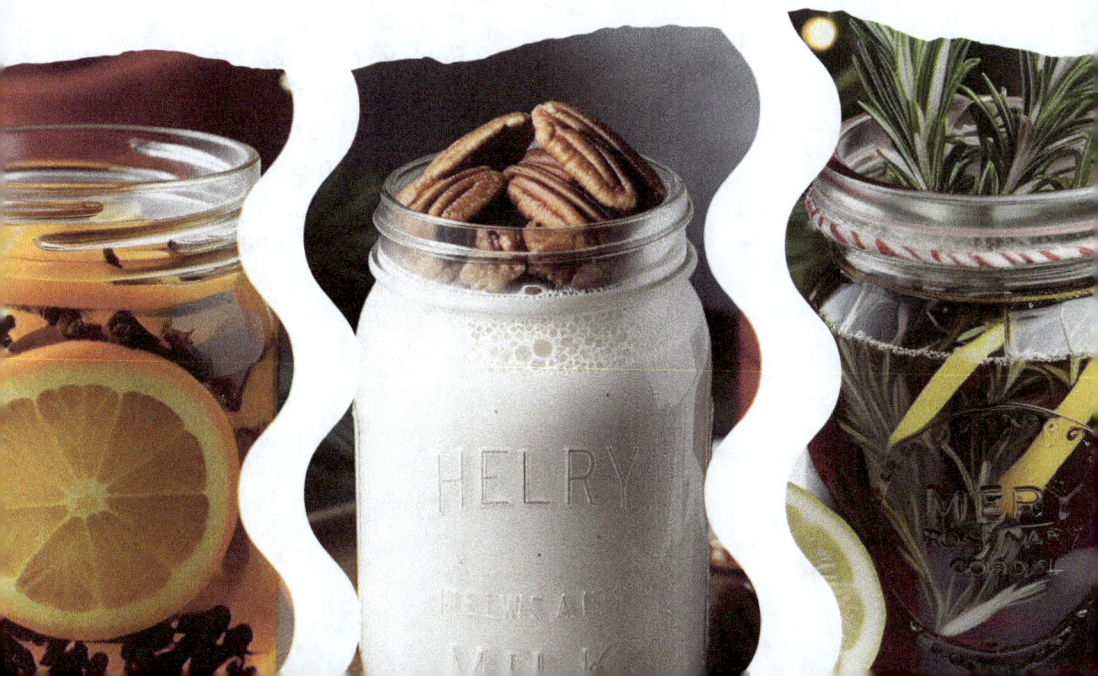

Cinnamon Syrup

Ingredients

- 1 cup water
- 1 cup granulated sugar
- 3 cinnamon sticks

Procedure

1. In a saucepan, combine the water, sugar, and cinnamon sticks.
2. Bring the mixture to a boil, then reduce the heat and simmer for 10 minutes.
3. Remove from heat and let the syrup steep for 15 minutes.
4. Strain out the cinnamon sticks and pour the syrup into a sterilized bottle or jar.
5. Store in the refrigerator for up to 2 weeks.

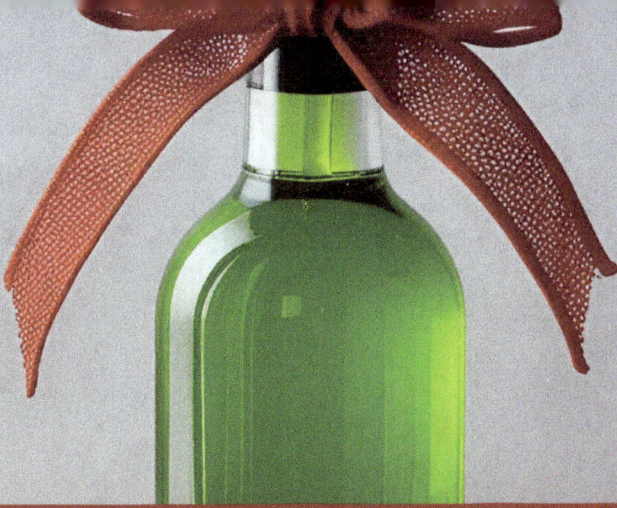

Peppermint Syrup

Ingredients

- 1 cup water
- 1 cup granulated sugar
- 1 cup fresh peppermint leaves

Procedure

1. In a saucepan, combine the water, sugar, and peppermint leaves.
2. Bring the mixture to a boil, then reduce the heat and simmer for 5 minutes.
3. Remove from heat and let the syrup steep for 15 minutes to infuse the peppermint flavor.
4. Strain out the leaves and pour the syrup into a sterilized bottle or jar.
5. Store in the refrigerator for up to 2 weeks.

Ginger Syrup

Ingredients

- 1 cup water
- 1 cup granulated sugar
- 1/2 cup fresh ginger root, sliced

Procedure

1. In a saucepan, combine the water, sugar, and ginger slices.
2. Bring the mixture to a boil, then reduce the heat and simmer for 10 minutes.
3. Remove from heat and let the syrup steep for 15 minutes.
4. Strain out the ginger slices and pour the syrup into a sterilized bottle or jar.
5. Store in the refrigerator for up to 2 weeks.

Rosemary Cordial

Ingredients

- 1 cup water
- 1 cup granulated sugar
- 3 sprigs fresh rosemary
- Zest of 1 lemon (optional for a citrus twist)

Procedure

1. In a saucepan, combine the water, sugar, rosemary sprigs, and lemon zest (if using).
2. Bring the mixture to a boil, then reduce the heat and simmer for 5 minutes.
3. Remove from heat and let it steep for 15 minutes.
4. Strain out the rosemary and zest, then pour the cordial into a sterilized bottle or jar.
5. Store in the refrigerator for up to 2 weeks.

Vanilla Bean Syrup

Ingredients

- 1 cup water
- 1 cup granulated sugar
- 1 vanilla bean, split

Procedure

1. In a saucepan, combine the water, sugar, and split vanilla bean.
2. Bring the mixture to a boil, then reduce the heat and simmer for 5 minutes.
3. Remove from heat and let the syrup steep for 15 minutes.
4. Remove the vanilla bean, then pour the syrup into a sterilized bottle or jar.
5. Store in the refrigerator for up to 2 weeks.

Pumpkin Spice Syrup

Ingredients

- 1 cup water
- 1 cup granulated sugar
- 2 tablespoons pumpkin puree
- 1/2 teaspoon ground cinnamon
- 1/4 teaspoon ground nutmeg
- 1/4 teaspoon ground cloves

Procedure

1. In a saucepan, combine the water, sugar, pumpkin puree, and spices.
2. Bring the mixture to a boil, then reduce the heat and simmer for 5 minutes.
3. Remove from heat and let the syrup cool slightly.
4. Strain through a fine mesh sieve to remove any solids, then pour the syrup into a sterilized bottle or jar.
5. Store in the refrigerator for up to 1 week.

Clove & Orange Infusion

Ingredients

- 1 cup water
- Zest of 1 orange
- 1 tablespoon whole cloves

Procedure

1. In a saucepan, combine water, orange zest, and cloves.
2. Bring the mixture to a boil, then reduce the heat and simmer for 5 minutes.
3. Remove from heat and let the infusion steep for 15 minutes.
4. Strain out the orange zest and cloves, then pour the infusion into a sterilized bottle or jar.

Maple Pecan Syrup

Ingredients

- 1 cup water
- 1/2 cup maple syrup
- 1/2 cup chopped toasted pecans

Procedure

1. In a saucepan, combine water, maple syrup, and chopped toasted pecans.
2. Bring the mixture to a boil, then reduce the heat and simmer for 10 minutes.
3. Remove from heat and let it steep for 15 minutes.
4. Strain out the pecans and pour the syrup into a sterilized bottle or jar.
5. Store in the refrigerator for up to 2 weeks.

Spiced Apple Cordial

Ingredients

- 1 cup fresh apple juice
- 1/2 cup water
- 1/2 cup granulated sugar
- 1 cinnamon stick
- 3 whole cloves
- 1 star anise

Procedure

1. In a saucepan, combine apple juice, water, sugar, and spices.
2. Bring the mixture to a boil, then reduce the heat and simmer for 10 minutes.
3. Remove from heat and let the cordial steep for 15 minutes.
4. Strain out the spices and pour the cordial into a sterilized bottle or jar.
5. Store in the refrigerator for up to 1 week.

Nutmeg Vanilla Infusion

Ingredients

- 1 cup water
- 1 cup granulated sugar
- 1 vanilla bean, split
- 1/2 teaspoon freshly grated nutmeg

Procedure

1. In a saucepan, combine water, sugar, vanilla bean, and grated nutmeg.
2. Bring the mixture to a boil, then reduce the heat and simmer for 5 minutes.
3. Remove from heat and let it steep for 15 minutes.
4. Strain out the vanilla bean and pour the infusion into a sterilized bottle or jar.
5. Store in the refrigerator for up to 2 weeks.

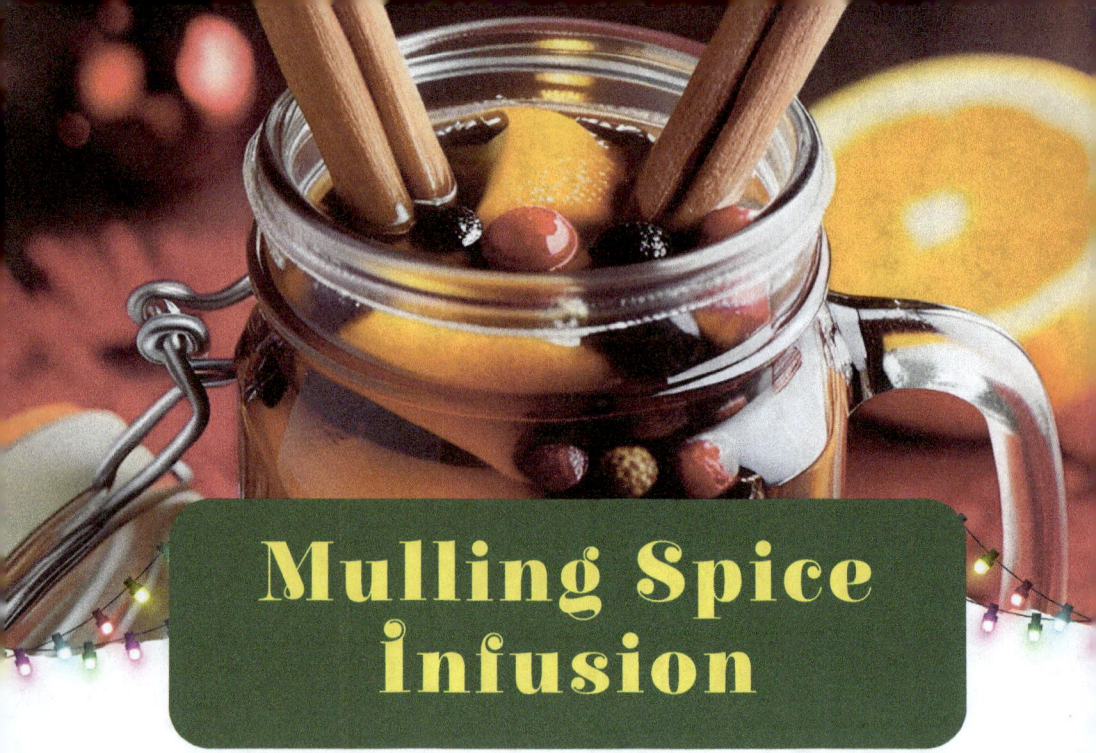

Mulling Spice Infusion

Ingredients

- 1 cup water
- 1 tablespoon mulling spices (cinnamon sticks, cloves, allspice berries, and star anise)
- Zest of 1 orange

Procedure

1. In a saucepan, combine water, mulling spices, and orange zest. Bring to a boil, then reduce the heat and simmer for 10 minutes.
2. Remove from heat and let the mixture steep for an additional 10 minutes.
3. Strain out the spices and pour the infusion into a sterilized bottle or jar. Store in the refrigerator for up to 2 weeks.

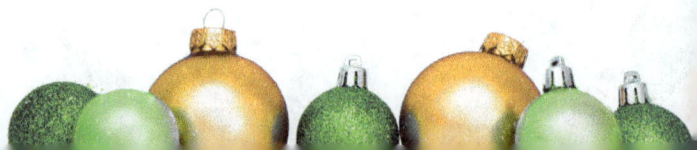

Pecan Milk

Ingredients

- 1 cup pecans (toasted)
- 4 cups water

Procedure

1. Toast the pecans in a dry skillet over medium heat for 3-5 minutes, until fragrant.
2. Blend the toasted pecans with water in a high-speed blender until smooth.
3. Strain the mixture through a nut milk bag or fine mesh sieve. Store in the refrigerator for up to 3 days.

Spiced Clove Syrup

Ingredients

- 1 cup water
- 1 cup granulated sugar
- 1 tablespoon whole cloves

Procedure

1. In a saucepan, combine water, sugar, and cloves. Bring to a boil, then reduce the heat and simmer for 5 minutes.
2. Remove from heat and let the syrup steep for 15 minutes.
3. Strain out the cloves and let the syrup cool before using.

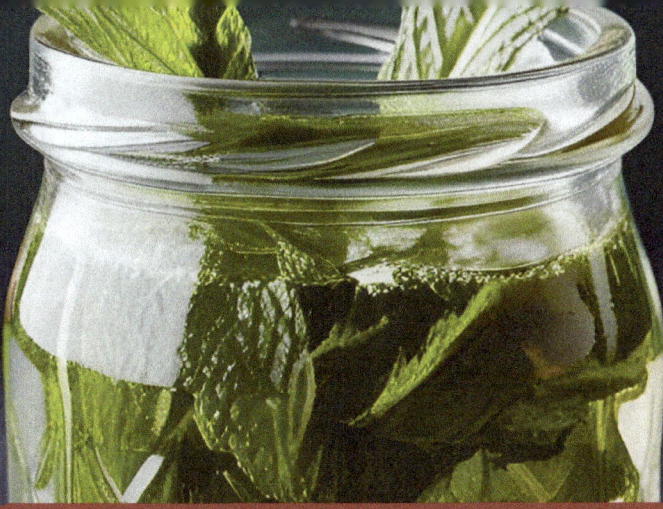

Mint Syrup

Ingredients

- 1 cup water
- 1 cup granulated sugar
- 1 cup fresh mint leaves

Procedure

1. In a saucepan, combine water, sugar, and mint leaves. Bring to a boil, then reduce the heat and simmer for 5 minutes.
2. Remove from heat and let the syrup steep for 15 minutes.
3. Strain out the mint leaves and let the syrup cool before using.

Thyme Syrup

Ingredients

- 1 cup water
- 1 cup granulated sugar
- 5 sprigs fresh thyme

Procedure

1. In a saucepan, combine water, sugar, and thyme sprigs. Bring to a boil, then reduce the heat and simmer for 5 minutes.
2. Remove from heat and let the mixture steep for 15 minutes.
3. Strain out the thyme and let the infusion cool before using.

Gingerbread Syrup

Ingredients

- 1 cup water
- 1 cup brown sugar
- 2 tablespoons molasses
- 1 teaspoon ground ginger
- 1 teaspoon ground cinnamon
- 1/4 teaspoon ground cloves
- 1/4 teaspoon ground nutmeg
- 1/2 teaspoon vanilla extract

Procedure

1. In a saucepan, combine water, brown sugar, molasses, ginger, cinnamon, cloves, and nutmeg.
2. Bring the mixture to a boil over medium heat, stirring until the sugar has fully dissolved.
3. Reduce the heat and let it simmer for 5-7 minutes, stirring occasionally.
4. Remove from heat and stir in the vanilla extract.
5. Let the syrup cool slightly, then pour it into a sterilized bottle or jar.
6. Store in the refrigerator for up to 3 weeks.

Basil Syrup

Ingredients

- 1 cup water
- 1 cup granulated sugar
- 1 cup fresh basil leaves

Procedure

1. In a saucepan, combine water, sugar, and basil leaves. Bring to a boil, then reduce the heat and simmer for 5 minutes.
2. Remove from heat and let the syrup steep for 15 minutes.
3. Strain out the basil leaves and let the syrup cool before using.

Caramel Syrup

Ingredients

- 1 cup water
- 1 cup granulated sugar
- 1/2 cup brown sugar
- 1/4 cup heavy cream

Procedure

1. In a saucepan, combine water, granulated sugar, and brown sugar. Bring to a boil, then reduce the heat and simmer for 10 minutes.
2. Remove from heat, then slowly stir in the cream. Let the syrup cool before using.

Orange Syrup

Ingredients

- 1 cup water
- 1 cup granulated sugar
- Zest of 1 orange, thinly peeled orange skin without the white pith attached.

Procedure

1. In a saucepan, combine water, sugar, and orange zest. Bring to a boil, then reduce the heat and simmer for 5 minutes.
2. Remove from heat and let the syrup cool before using.

Stay Cozy, Stay Connected!

Thank you so much for choosing *Mocktails for the Holidays!* We hope these festive drinks bring a little extra sparkle to your celebrations and joy to every glass you pour.

If you loved this book, we'd be so grateful if you could take a moment to leave a review on Amazon. Your feedback helps others discover our books —and it means the world to independent creators like us.

To make things easy, just scan the QR code below or visit **greensaucepublishing.com**

From there, you can:

- **Leave a review** on Amazon
- **Discover the other books** in the Mocktails for Every Day series
- **Join our mailing list** for updates, freebies, and new releases
- **Follow us** on social media and join the conversation

We'd love to see your creations! Tag us with your favorite mocktails or holiday moments using *#MocktailsForEveryDay*.

Wishing you a season full of joy, warmth, and beautiful alcohol-free moments.

Cheers from all of us at Green Sauce Publishing!

The Green Sauce Publishing Team

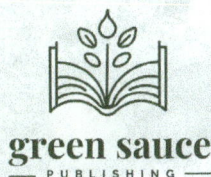

green sauce
— PUBLISHING —

ALSO AVAILABLE, GET THE WHOLE SERIES!

Mocktails for the Holidays is the sixth book in our **Mocktails for Every Day Series.** Check out the other books in the series, already published, or coming soon, by scanning the QR Code on page 85!

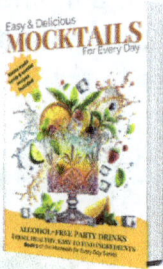

Easy & Delicious Mocktails for Every Day

Explore a world of vibrant, alcohol-free cocktails that prove fun and sophistication don't require spirits. Using fresh, easy-to-find ingredients, you'll craft party-ready drinks, from fruity infusions to zesty syrups.

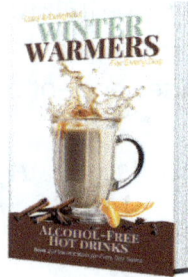

Cozy & Delightful Winter Warmers

Warm and Cozy, comforting and delicious. Our Winter Warmers are just perfect for long Winter evenings or cozy Winter mornings, or any occasion with friends and family.

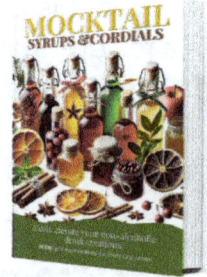

Mocktail Syrups & Cordials

All our homemade syrups, cordials and infusions gathered together in one beautiful book. Use our syrups in any drinks, or gift them to your friends and family

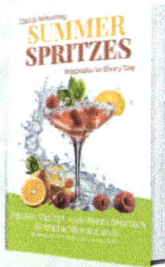

Cool & Refreshing Summer Spritzes Mocktails for Every Day

Thirst quenching, beautiful and delicious. Our Summer Spritzes are the perfect alcohol-free accompaniment for any occasion, for anyone.

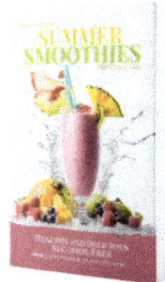

Dairy-Free Summer Smoothies

Deliciously creamy, but 100% Dairy Free, our Delicious Dairy-Free Summer Smoothies will take your summer mornings to the next level!

www.ingramcontent.com/pod-product-compliance
Lightning Source LLC
LaVergne TN
LVHW022341080426
835508LV00012BA/1303